The Impact of Health Care

Michael Welker | Eva Winkler | John Witte, Jr.
Stephen Pickard (Eds.)

The Impact of Health Care

on Character Formation, Ethical Education,
and the Communication of Values
in Late Modern Pluralistic Societies

WIPF & STOCK · Eugene, Oregon

Wipf and Stock Publishers
199 W 8th Ave, Suite 3
Eugene, OR 97401

The Impact of Health Care
On Character Formation, Ethical Education, and the Communication
of Values in Late Modern Pluralistic Societies
By Welker, Michael and Winkler, Eva
Copyright © 2023 Evangelische Verlagsanstalt GmbH All rights reserved.
Softcover ISBN-13: 978-1-6667-8059-8
Hardcover ISBN-13: 978-1-6667-8060-4
Publication date 5/22/2023
Previously published by Evangelische Verlagsanstalt GmbH, 2023

Table of Contents

Acknowledgments 7

Preface to the Series 9

Eva C. Winkler and Michael Welker
Introduction 13

PART ONE: MEDICAL ETHICS BETWEEN MEDICINE AND ECONOMY

Eva C. Winkler
Time for a New Oath? The Role of the Individual Physician's Ethos and Institutional Ethics in the Face of Economization of the Health-Care System 23

Günter Thomas
Mercy under Conditions of Scarcity and the Need for Organization; or, Where Is the Humane Ethos Located in the Health-Care System? An Outline of the Problem 35

Christine Thomas
Ethical Tensions in the Medical Treatment of Elderly Patients in Geriatrics and Geriatric Psychiatry 45

PART TWO: ETHICAL IMPACTS OF ADVANCING MEDICAL RESEARCH AND TECHNIQUES

Anthony D. Ho
The Impact of Advances in Stem Cell and Genome Research on Ethical Decision-Making 53

Ruth M. Farrell
The Acceptance of Genetic Technologies by Individuals, Societies, and Health-Care Systems 65

Karla Alex and Eva C. Winkler
Ethical Discourse on Epigenetics and Genome Editing: The Risk of (Epi-)Genetic Determinism and Scientifically Controversial Basic Assumptions 77

Andreas Unterberg and Pavlina Lenga
The Impact of Advances in Surgical Techniques and Quality-of-Life Considerations on Ethical Decision-Making and Education in Neurosurgery 101

PART THREE: DIGITAL MEDICINE AND ETHICAL DECISIONS

Giovanni Rubeis and Nadia Primc
Ethical Aspects of Digital Transformation in Medicine and Health Care   121

Beate Ditzen and Christian P. Schaaf
Family Decision-Making in Times of Genomic Newborn Screening   137

PART FOUR: HEALTH CARE: HISTORY, EDUCATION, PRACTICE

Karen Nolte
On the History of the Nursing Ethos in Germany   153

Thorsten Moos
Health-Care Chaplains and Medical Ethics: Clinical and Educational Experiences   165

Gregor Etzelmüller
Medical Anthropology and Theology on Human Destiny   175

Peter Kirsch
Psychotherapy, Personality, and the Role of Values   197

Contributors   203

Acknowledgments

A consultation leading to this volume took place at the Forschungszentrum Internationale und Interdisziplinäre Theologie (FIIT) at the University of Heidelberg in April 2022. We are most grateful to the McDonald Agape Foundation and President Peter McDonald for the generous support of the consultation and this publication.

We thank Gary S. Hauk for his careful editing of the texts and the publishing houses Evangelische Verlangsanstalt in Leipzig and Wipf & Stock in Eugene, Oregon, for their good cooperation.

Michael Welker and Eva C. Winkler

Preface to the Series

Five hundred years ago, Protestant reformer Martin Luther argued that "three estates" (drei Stände) lie at the foundation of a just and orderly society—marital families, religious communities, and political authorities. Parents in the home; pastors in the church; magistrates in the state—these, said Luther, are the three authorities whom God appointed to represent divine justice and mercy in the world, to protect peace and liberty in earthly life. Household, church, and state—these are the three institutional pillars on which to build social systems of education and schooling, charity and social welfare, economy and architecture, art and publication. Family, faith, and freedom—these are the three things that people will die for.

In the half millennium since Luther, historians have uncovered various classical and Christian antecedents to these early Protestant views. Numerous later theorists have propounded all manner of variations and applications of this three-estates theory, many increasingly abstracted from Luther's overtly Christian worldview. Early modern covenant theologians, both Christian and Jewish, described the marital, confessional, and political covenants that God calls human beings to form, each directed to interrelated personal and public ends. Social-contract theorists differentiated the three contracts that humans enter as they move from the state of nature to an organized society protective of their natural rights—the marital contract of husband and wife; the government contract of rulers and citizens; and, for some, the religious contracts of preachers and parishioners. Early anthropologists posited three stages of development of civilization—from family-based tribes and clans, to priest-run theocracies, to fully organized states that embraced all three institutions. Sociologists distinguished three main forms of authority in an organized community: "traditional" authority that begins in the home, "charismatic" authority that is exemplified by the church, and "legal" authority that is rooted in the state. Legal historians outlined three stages of development of legal norms—from the habits and rules of the family, to the customs and canons of religion, to the statutes and codes of the state.

Already a century ago, however, scholars in different fields began to flatten out this hierarchical theory of social institutions and to emphasize the foundational role of other social institutions alongside the family, church, and state in shaping private and public life and character. Sociologists like Max Weber and Talcott Parsons emphasized the shaping powers of "technical rationality" exemplified especially in new industry, scientific education, and market economies. Legal scholars like Otto von Gierke and F. W. Maitland emphasized the critical roles of nonstate legal associations (*Genossenschaften*) in maintaining a just social, political, and legal order historically and today. Catholic subsidiarity theories of Popes Leo XIII and Pius XI emphasized the essential task of mediating social units between the individual and the state to cater the full range of needs, interests, rights, and duties of individuals. Protestant theories of sphere sovereignty, inspired by Abraham Kuyper, argued that not only churches, states, and families but also the social spheres of art, labor, education, economics, agriculture, recreation, and more should enjoy a level of independence from others, especially an overreaching church or state. Various theories of social or structural pluralism, civil society, voluntary associations, the independent sector, multiculturalism, multinormativity, and other such labels have now come to the fore in the ensuing decades—both liberal and conservative, religious and secular, and featuring all manner of methods and logics.

Pluralism of all sorts is now a commonplace of late modern societies. At minimum, this means a multitude of free and equal individuals and a multitude of groups and institutions, each with very different political, moral, religious, and professional interests and orientations. It includes the sundry associations, interest groups, parties, lobbies, and social movements that often rapidly flourish and fade around a common cause, especially when aided by modern technology and various social media. Some see in this texture of plurality an enormous potential for colorful and creative development and a robust expression of human and cultural freedom. Others see a chaotic individualism and radical relativism, which endangers normative education, moral character formation, and effective cultivation of enduring values or virtues.

Pluralism viewed as vague plurality, however, focuses on only one aspect of late modern societies—the equality of individuals, and their almost unlimited freedom to participate peaceably at any time as a respected voice in the moral reasoning and civil interactions of a society. But this view does not adequately recognize that, beneath the shifting diversity of social forms and norms that constitute modernity, pluralistic societies have heavy normative codes that shape their individual and collective values and morals, preferences and prejudices.

The sources of much of this normative coding and moral education in late modern pluralistic societies are the deep and powerful social systems that are the pillars of every advanced culture. The most powerful and pervasive of these are the social systems of law, religion, politics, science/academy, market, media, family, education, medicine, and national defense. The actual empirical forms of each of these powerful social systems can and do vary greatly, even in the relatively homogeneous societies of the late modern West. But these deeper social systems in one form or another are structurally essential and often normatively decisive in individual and communal lives.

Every advanced society has a comprehensive legal system of justice and order, religious systems of ritual and doctrine, a family system of procreation and love, an economic system of trade and value, a media system of communication and dissemination of news and information, and an educational system of creation, preservation, and application of knowledge and scientific advance. Many advanced societies also have massive systems of science, technology, health care, and national defense with vast influence over and through all of these other social systems. These pervasive social systems lie at the foundation of modern advanced societies, and they anchor the vast pluralities of associations and social interactions that might happen to exist at any given time.

Each of these social systems has internal value systems, institutionalized rationalities, and normative expectations that together help to shape each individual's morality and character. Each of these social spheres, moreover, has its own professionals and experts who shape and implement its internal structures and processes. The normative network created by these social spheres is often harder to grasp today, since late modern pluralistic societies usually do not bring these different value systems to light under the dominance of just one organization, institution, and power. And this normative network has also become more shifting and fragile, especially since traditional social systems, such as religion and the family, have eroded in their durability and power, and other social systems, such as science, the market, healthcare, defense, and the media, have become more powerful.

The aim of this project on "Character Formation and Ethical Education in Late Modern Pluralistic Societies" is to identify the realities and potentials of these core social systems to provide moral orientation and character formation in our day. What can and should these social spheres, separately and together, do in shaping the moral character of late modern individuals who, by nature, culture, and constitutional norms, are free and equal in dignity and rights? What are and should be the core educational functions and moral responsibilities of each of these social spheres? How can we better understand and better influence the complex interactions among individualism, the normative binding powers of these social systems, and the creativity of civil groups and institutions? How can we map and measure the different hierarchies of values that govern each of these social systems, and that are also interwoven and interconnected in various ways in shaping late modern understandings of the common good? How do we negotiate the boundaries and conflicts between and among these social systems when one encroaches on the other, or imposes its values and rationalities on individuals at the cost of the other social spheres or of the common good? What and where are the intrinsic strengths of each social sphere that should be made more overt in character formation, public education, and the shaping of minds and mentalities?

These are some of the guiding questions at work in this project and in this volume. Our project aims to provide a systematic account of the role of these powerful normative codes operating in the social spheres of law, religion, the family, the market, the media, science and technology, the academy, health care, and military and defense systems in the late modern liberal West. Our focus is on selected examples and case studies drawn from Western Europe, North America, South Africa, and Australia, which together provide just enough diversity to test out broader theories of character formation and moral education. Our scholars are drawn from across the academy, with representative voices from the humanities, social sciences, and natural sciences as well as the professions of theology, law, business, and medicine. While most of our scholars come from the Protestant and Catholic worlds, our endeavor is to offer comparative insights that will help scholars from any profession or confession. While our laboratory is principally Western liberal societies, the modern forces of globalization will soon make these issues of moral character formation a concern for every culture and region of the world—given the power of global social media, entertainment, and sports; the pervasiveness of global finance, business, trade, and law; and the perennial global worries over food, health care, environmental degradation, and natural disasters.

In this volume, we focus in on the role of health care and health-care systems in shaping character development, ethical education, and the communication of values in late modern pluralistic societies.

Michael Welker, University of Heidelberg
Eva C. Winkler, University of Heidelberg
John Witte Jr., Emory University
Stephen Pickard, Charles Sturt University

Introduction

Eva C. Winkler and Michael Welker

This volume focuses on the role of health care and medicine in their impact on character formation, ethical education, and the communication of values in late modern pluralistic societies. The contributions are arranged in four sections. The first deals with the tensions that medical ethics faces between the demands of medical ethos and the challenges of the economization of health care. The second part addresses ethical impacts of advancing medical research and techniques. The third part looks at some ethical aspects of the digital transformation in medicine and health care. The fourth part is concerned with developments in ethos and education in health care and medicine, with different perspectives on human destiny in medical anthropology and theology, and with a view of psychotherapy on the topics of the volume.

Part One addresses the ethical tensions in the health-care system between professional responsibilities toward the individual patient and realizing those responsibilities in a complex health-care system with limited resources.

Eva C. Winkler sets out to define the role of professional ethics for the individual doctor as well as derived desiderata for organizational ethics in the face of economization of the health-care system in Germany, where financial pressure has increased in recent years. She reports the empirical data indicating that the so-called economization has significant impact on medical decision-making and action and consequently potentially also on the doctor–patient relationship. While economic considerations are necessary and in part desired—for example, when the same goal can be achieved by less expensive means—other economic incentives can compromise the quality of treatment and trust in the entire medical profession.

She starts with the physician's perspective on economic incentives reflected in empirical data and then analyzes three different responses to cost pressure from a normative perspective with considerations about the appropriate forms of economization in the medical system: enhancing efficiency, increasing revenue, and rationing or forgoing effective medical interventions to save money. She then evaluates the types of ethical guidance available to physicians to resolve tensions between their mission to ensure their patients' welfare, on one hand, and their responsibility for cost-conscious decisions, on the other. Finally, she illuminates the limitations of "appeals to individual ethos" and personal responsibility, and she discusses the necessary embedding of the individual in institutional ethics and the importance of decision-making above the patient-physician level. She then proposes potential guardrails for ethical decision-making in view of cost considerations.

Günter Thomas begins with reflections on the theological-historical background of an ethos of caring for the sick in Christianity and beyond. This ethos has often been considered in frameworks of person-to-person relations. This orientation, however, has to be re-investigated today with respect to the social distribution of values in health-care organizations. Thomas names the complex network of medical institutions, health insurers, public or government funding of health care, the ethos of human actors and clinical staff, and the various expectations of patients. How to orchestrate this complex network with its differing value systems of orientation and the associated expectations? How to deal with the problem that "organized communities of solidarity must always be inclusive and exclusive at the same time in order to function effectively"?

Thomas concludes with considerations on "orientational distress." He asks for religious, academic, and civil-societal contexts in which broader visions of a good, fulfilled, and successful life can be discussed "without damaging the latent protection in the health-care organization itself." He argues for intensified discourses between those who deal with religiously and ethically based value orientation and those who deal with the ethical and practical challenges of health care in order to reduce orientational distress and prevent eventual burnout.

Christine Thomas specifies such challenges with respect to the medical treatment of elderly patients. She describes conflicts over a patient's sovereignty of interpretation and decision-making, conflicts between patients and their relatives or younger generations, and conflicts also between patients and families, on one hand, and medical and therapeutic practitioners, on the other. A broad spectrum of potential problems arises, from unrealistic demands for maximum therapy to a resigned "nihilism" of frail patients or a laissez-faire attitude on the part of the patient or relatives, but also from limitations in hospital financing and mental and physical capacities of the medical and nursing staff.

She pleads to uphold the demands of ethical responsibility and a community of solidarity, to "return to the principle of no harm" in medical practice and to "initiatives such as 'choosing wisely'" between overmedication and underuse. She also argues for "targeted face-to-face communication between treatment providers and patients" and the eventual "moderation of an ethics adviser."

Part Two of this book turns to ethical challenges that come with advancing medical research and techniques.

Anthony D. Ho uses the powerful tool of storytelling and shares stories of cancer patients to illustrate situations that call for ethical considerations. The first story raises questions about how far a patient with terminal disease should be encouraged to undergo experimental treatments with unknown risks, and it highlights the inherent tension between palliative care and early-phase clinical studies for advancing science. The second is a success story about a patient who also received a new and experimental treatment—a stem cell transplantation—and raises ethical questions about the balance between individual health needs and community resource allocation, the financial gains of expensive medical procedures, and the justified price of a novel product or profit margin for the pharmaceutical industry. The third story highlights the detrimental impact of premature communication of not-yet consolidated scientific advances on clinical decision-making and concludes that properly conducted research is paramount to establish robust evidence and efficacy of novel treatments. As an example of successful regulation, the chapter portrays the development of the German Stem Cell Act—a regulation that permits scientific advances under ethical considerations. With these stories, Ho highlights not only the character formation required for proper interaction with patients, but also the ethical challenges that arise as medical technology advances, and he underscores the need for ongoing ethical education and communication of values in the health-care system.

Ruth M. Farrell reports on advances in genomic science and technology that have had an impact on reproductive health care, particularly prenatal care, where genetic tests can inform decisions about reproductive health and family building. However, the complexity and uncertainty of genomic information before birth present challenges for patients, families, and society. Prenatal genetic tests can inform significant decisions during pregnancy, including the possibility of ending the pregnancy if a serious condition is diagnosed. Farrell draws a very nuanced picture. On one hand, it is important that decisions about the use of genetic testing reflect the values, needs, and goals of pregnant women and their families. On the other hand, these decisions are also embedded and thus influenced by social systems, which impact actionability and agency during pregnancy, with significant ramifications for individuals, families, communities, and future generations.

Farrell illustrates the various spheres of influence that determine agency: first, the ability to access genetic testing and to process and interpret the information about genetic test results, but also the options provided to act upon the information and decide whether to end a pregnancy. She not only raises concerns about a woman's ability to access abortion services in the United States if a severe fetal genetic condition is identified. She also considers whether a medical condition perceived as dysfunction is not only a matter of science but also in part socially determined and dependent upon the social infrastructure that enables differently abled individuals to interact within their families and communities. Hence, she illustrates how scientific development is influenced by societal values, which establish parameters for the acceptable uses of technology.

Karla Alex and *Eva C. Winkler* write about new developments in genetics and epigenetics research, and take a look at scientifically and ethically contested conceptions that form the ethical, scientific, and popular scientific discourse. The chapter includes two tables that concisely summarize the new research techniques of epigenome editing and genome editing, as well as several -isms and their respective discourse areas. Theses -isms are conceptions about the impact of genetics and epigenetics on a person's (and potentially their descendants') life and associated responsibilities for health. Alex and Winkler keenly scrutinize and critically assess these conceptions.

Building on this analysis, they compare the ethical debate on genome editing with the ethical debate on epigenetics. They show that the concept of genetic determinism might be indirectly present in contemporary discussions on genome editing. Likewise, they note how notions of epigenetic determinism are present across scientific, ethical, and popular scientific discourse, especially in the form of the presumption of heritability of epigenetic information acquired during life. The authors point out that this presumption is at best scientifically contested (if not unproven) for humans, a fact that is beginning to be acknowledged in ethical discourse, with a resulting shift of focus in epigenetics discourse from individual responsibilities to social and environmental justice at a population level. In conclusion, they argue that concepts like genetic and epigenetic determinism "are increasingly viewed critically in ethical discourse because they cannot be confirmed scientifically. In popular scientific debates in particular, however, they seem to persist, which ultimately also influences the public discussion. Since a broad public discussion is required especially for genome editing, a reflective handling of the different -isms analyzed in this chapter is central."

Andreas Unterberg and Pavlina Lenga examine the implications of technological advances in surgery that have led to the challenge of sub- or superspecialization. They set out by compiling the inventory that is necessary for a neurosurgeon nowadays to maneuver the choppy waters of ethical challenges: professionalism and a pledge to put the patient's interest first; transparency and awareness of conflicts of interest with the pharmaceutical or technical-device industry; shared decision-making oriented toward the patient's goals and values; and education that sensitizes neurosurgical trainees to the ethical dimensions of their daily work.

The authors highlight the four midlevel principles of medical ethics (respect for autonomy, beneficence, nonmaleficence, and justice) as guardrails for such ethical evaluation. They exemplify the weighing of quality of life, survival time, and other patient-oriented factors by using three different disease scenarios. The first presents glioblastoma as a very aggressive brain tumor that affects the patient's quality of life significantly, while surgery can restore quality of life. The second scenario describes the course of benign tumors, such as craniopharyngiomas, where surgical resection can lead to worsened quality of life. In the third case, age-related degenerative changes can affect the spinal elements, leading to neurogenic claudication or lumbar radiculopathy and a decrease in mobility and quality of life, where there is no clear consensus on the optimal treatment for octogenarians, although surgery even in very old and frail patients can be beneficial.

In Part Three, we turn to some ethical aspects connected with the digital transformation of medicine and health care.

The seminal contribution by *Giovanni Rubeis and Nadia Primc* aims to overcome confusions and worries connected with the "umbrella concept of digital transformation," which covers automation, mechanization, machinization, robotization, and data-driven technologies, and is promoted by different academic disciplines and stakeholders with very different perspectives and interests. How can a "digital disruption of health care" be avoided and a "process of incremental change and (intended) improvement of health care" through digital technologies be envisioned?

The chapter identifies three criteria for positive developments:
- emphasis on the autonomy of patients in the form of their participation in the treatment process, and the critical evaluation of factors that hinder empowerment;
- differentiating technologies that support autonomy from technologies that risk the well-being of patients;
- investigation of the introduction of nonhuman actors into the clinical encounter with the question whether they support or minimize "the willingness of patients to trust health professionals."

After pondering open questions of "justice and inequalities in digitalized health care," the chapter identifies helpful strategies to promote digital transformation: a participatory technological design; transparency of "parameters of an algorithm-based system"; and a continuous improvement of "health-care literacy." It concludes with a call for "respect of the autonomy of patients, the promotion of well-being of patients, and the prevention of inequalities between patients."

Beate Ditzen and Christian P. Schaaf anticipate yet another important advancement in medicine—genetic newborn screening. Genetic newborn screening is a process that can identify specific diseases in newborns that require early intervention to improve health or save lives. Predictive genetic testing is also available for families with a history of childhood-onset disorders, where preventive interventions are available. The authors report on the factors that are important for individuals and families during and following genetic testing in general and the lessons learned in the pilot projects on genomic newborn screening. Apart from the ambivalence about uptake of genetic testing with a known "intention-behavior-gap," the authors address challenges that might become exacerbated with genomic newborn screening: dealing with the uncertainty of genetic predictions, the challenge to comprehend probability scores and their implications for action, and different coping styles in dealing with risk information.

The authors suggest concrete communication strategies for explaining false positive results and variants of unknown significance, as well as metrics for communicating actionable results along five dimensions: severity, likelihood, efficacy of intervention, burden of intervention, and knowledge base. The authors suggest that dyadic decision models can help identify parameters that predict whether couples will decide to use genomic testing and, if so, how they will wish the results to be communicated. Decision aids can ease decision-making in a complex and value-based medical context, where stress levels can impair processing and memory of important information. Therefore, the ways in which information is presented to parents, as well as the timing and context of decision-making, are crucial factors. The authors hint of a forthcoming research project where they will investigate these factors to set up a framework that allows for the benefits of early intervention on genomic screening but prevents potential stigmatization and negative sequelae.

The contributions in Part Four of this volume present case studies of ethical problems in history, in education, and in the praxis of health care, as well as outside perspectives on it.

Karen Nolte shows that the current smoldering crisis of the nursing profession has become most acute with the COVID-19 pandemic. She looks back on the long period of work on the nursing ethos in Germany since 1782. It started with books by physicians who tried to combine an ethos of self-sacrificial love in favor of the sick and the poor with the establishment of nursing as a medical auxiliary activity.

"Good training in nursing should serve to combat illness as well as poverty, including spiritual poverty." Against the widespread view in Germany that nurses should be "devoted and obedient," Florence Nightingale formulated a secular nursing ethos with a strong medical emphasis. She spoke of an "intelligent obedience" to the "head nurses," whereas German authors talked about unconditional obedience to the doctors.

Up to the middle of the twentieth century, nursing in Germany was organized in sisterhoods, most of them connected with Christian denominations. When, in the middle of the century, "fewer and fewer young women were willing to give up a private life and family," Germany started recruiting nursing staff from southern European countries, and later from Asia. When municipalities that had covered most of the costs of their hospitals could no longer afford to finance hospital budgets, a complex crisis of the nursing system became apparent. The attempt to combat it through functional nursing, which split responsibilities among nurses, led to an increased crisis and calls for better patient-oriented care and "holistic nursing." Although a Christian nursing ethos is still present today, "most nurses emphasize their professionalism and demand appropriate recognition of their work and adequate pay."

Thorsten Moos, in his chapter, explains why "ethics in the clinic has experienced a boom in recent decades." Several contributions to this book emphasize the tremendous importance of not only respect for patient autonomy, but also mental, psychological, and therapeutic limits in dealing with a questionable "free will" of persons in life-threatening situations. Sensitivity to the limits of pastoral care as religious and psychological communication, on one hand, and "a narrowing of medical ethics towards a decision-making technique in difficult treatments," on the other, has led to strong investments in pastoral-care education and a new climate of integration of hospital chaplains in dealing with the complex fields of interaction between physicians and patients, relatives and next generations, and clinical staff and all sorts of counseling voices.

Moos emphasizes the potential of pastoral competence in dealing with different ethical convictions, not only among patients but also among clinical staff. He argues that "ethical competence in clinical pastoral care encompasses more than a set of *additional* knowledge and skills" complementing "'old' pastoral tools." He stresses the complicated but morally highly valuable goal of giving "the patient a voice in the conflict between doctors and relatives" and, in situations of deep personal distress and great difficulties, in articulating their own will.

Gregor Etzelmüller introduces the human search for "health" beyond the experience of physical healing. He works with Viktor von Weizsäcker's insight that patients "challenge physicians to expand the boundaries of their professional expertise" by asking "for the destiny of their lives." He also relates to basic insights of the Apostle Paul that the bodily, mental, and conscious existence of human beings is directed toward a destiny to experience love and hope and faith, and to communicate these gifts of the Spirit to others. Etzelmüller's own work in the interdisciplinary discourse on "embodied cognition" and the focus of Weizsäcker and Paul on "the wisdom of the lived body" and the complex roles of illness provide a framework for the contribution.

Weizsäcker argued that "the disease needs to be understood in the entirety of the person's life," that "every illness has a meaning," and he called for a search to reorient one's life. Paul frequently reflected on the interdependence of individual illness and suffering and the life in the community in which the sick individual lives. It is not only important to gain an understanding of what the sick body wants to communicate beyond pain and malfunctioning. The edifying gifts of the Spirit (in the light of the law: justice, mercy, and the search for truth; in the light of the gospel: love, hope, and faith) have to be discerned and strengthened in the communication between the community and the individual, between the individuals and the community.

Etzelmüller adds the voices of Heidegger, Whitehead, Barth, Arendt, Nussbaum, and others in order to explore resources that might help in this task. The human conscience and a self-critical stance toward it, the escape from the "spell of the 'they' (*das Man*)," and finding the "right balance between self-effacement und vitality" all are brought into focus.

The final chapter, by *Peter Kirsch*, begins with the helpful definition of personality as "the totality of all temporally stable characteristics of a person, which determine his or her experience and behavior." Kirsch adds the classic definition of psychotherapy by Johannes Strotzka: a "deliberate and planned interactional process for influencing behavioral disturbances and states of suffering deemed by consensus to require treatment ... by psychological means ... toward a defined goal ... worked out together ... by means of teachable techniques based on a theory of normal and pathological behavior."

Kirsch stresses the complexities of "personality disorders" in various conflicts among four different basic needs (the needs "for orientation and control," "for pleasure and avoidance of displeasure," for attachment, and for self-esteem). The great challenges of psychotherapy lie in the difficulty of helping people become aware of their "basic needs, values, and resulting goals for action." Psychotherapy has to avoid paternalistic approaches and has to take the patient's autonomy and self-determination seriously. It reaches its limits when the goals of the patient "are contrary to the fundamental values of our society or of the therapist."

In sum, the contributions to this volume offer a wide range of challenges to medical ethics. There are the tensions between the individual physician's ethos and the stresses of the economization of the health-care system. Many conflicts of expectations and needs in the complex network of medical institutions with human actors and clinical staff, the realms of health insurers and public or governmental funding of health care, and various expectations of patients and relatives all have to be considered. Adding to the complexity are tensions between patient autonomy and sovereignty of decision-making and the insight into therapeutic needs by medical practitioners, and tensions between expectations of maximum therapy and patients' sometimes stubborn will to resignation.

Helpful developments in new forms of education in medical ethics and a better cooperation among different actors in medical treatment and hospital care are sadly correlated with a complicated history of nursing, with various forms of lack of respect and economic exploitation. Deeper visions of human health and illusionary and counterproductive perceptions of the individual and the common good in health care have to be discerned.

Part One:
Medical Ethics Between Medicine and Economy

Time for a New Oath? The Role of the Individual Physician's Ethos and Institutional Ethics in the Face of Economization of the Health-Care System

Eva C. Winkler

The topic of economization in the health-care system has been rampant for many years, but has been gaining momentum in Germany since 2018 in particular, with a number of wake-up calls. The Association of the Scientific Medical Societies in Germany (AWMF) published an action paper against the undue influence of economic interests on medical decisions.[1] The popular magazine *Der Stern* published an urgent request against the economization of German hospitals that was signed by numerous medical associations, specialist societies, individual doctors, and well-known medical ethicists.[2] And in 2021, at the annual meeting of the German Medical Association, the delegates overwhelmingly supported the proposal against commercialization in the health-care system made by the board of directors of the German Medical Association (BÄK), saying, "The medical profession rejects performance, financial, resource, and behavioral requirements that affect responsible medical practice and are incompatible with medical ethics."[3]

These appeals speak to the dilemma that many physicians face—on one hand, the mandate to provide a standard of care and contribute to the well-being of their patients, and on the other hand, the need to be held responsible for their own department, clinical practice, or hospital to be economically balanced or even to generate revenues. The debate also shows that the term "economization" is used to mean everything from practices of increasing efficiency to a primary profit orientation in health care.

---

[1] AWMF, "Medizin und Ökonomie–Maßnahmen für eine wissenschaftlich begründete, patientenzentrierte und ressourcenbewusste Versorgung."

[2] "Der Ärzteappel–gegen die Diktatur der Ökonomie in unseren Krankenhäusern," *Der Stern*, no. 37, Sep. 5, 2019.

[3] *Deutsches Ärzteblatt*, Nov. 2, 2021, "Ärztetag lehnt Kommerzialisierung ab," https://www.aerzteblatt.de/nachrichten/128581/Aerztetag-lehnt-Kommerzialisierung-ab-aerztliches-Handeln-muss-unbeeinflusst-bleiben.

In this chapter, I use the term to describe a process in which the logic of medical decisions is possibly influenced through economic goals and modes of action.[4] That is, the concept of economization is used descriptively and value-neutrally. It can therefore indicate ethically positive as well as negative consequences of such an economic influence on the medical logic of action.

One example of the positive effects of economic considerations in medical practice is the rationalization of work steps to optimize the time/result ratio without negatively impacting the quality of patient care. Examples of negative effects include the performance of procedures that are not medically indicated due to financial incentives, or forgoing medically indicated measures in order to save costs (rationing). Different degrees of economization can be distinguished. Accordingly, both contexts in which cost considerations play no role at all and those in which costs do play a decisive role are conceivable in the extreme forms, as are contexts in which a profit must be made in any case.[5]

Reasons for Economization and Empirical Data on Economic Influences in Health Care

The background reasons for the increasing economization in the German medical system are manifold. The drivers of rising costs are longer life expectancy and rising therapeutical costs. Against the background of limited resources, health-care expenditures have been regulated in recent years and decades by a variety of political and legal instruments. One example of this is the financing of inpatient care introduced in 2004 through the G-DRG system (German version of the Diagnoses Related Groups reporting and reimbursement system), which has also been studied with regard to its possible effects on care.[6] Physicians and other health-care professionals have repeatedly pointed out that the financial pressures on the German medical system have increased in recent years, and that the so-called economization has considerable consequences for medical de-

---

[4] Heiner Raspe, "Indikationsstellung in der klinischen Medizin: Dem Individuum und/oder dem Patientenkollektiv verpflichtet?," *Medizinrecht* 34, no. 4 (2016): 248–50, DOI: 10.1007/s00350-016-4244-y.

[5] Arne Manzeschke, "Die effiziente Organisation," *Ethik in der Medizin* 23, no. 4 (2011): 271–82.

[6] Bernard Braun et al., *Pauschalpatienten, Kurzlieger und Draufzahler. Auswirkungen der DRGs auf Versorgungsqualität und Arbeitsbedingungen im Krankenhaus* (Bern: Huber, 2010); and Antonius Reifferscheid, Dominik Thomas, and Jürgen Wasem, "Zehn Jahre DRG-System in Deutschland–Theoretische Anreizwirkungen und empirische Evidenz," *Krankenhaus-Report 2013* (Stuttgart: Schattauer, 2013), 3–19.

cision-making and actions.⁷ The influence of financial incentives on physician decision-making has been empirically investigated in a few studies in recent years. Exemplary of this are data indicating that medical interventions and measures are adapted to the possibilities for billing.⁸ Economic factors are also described by physicians as relevant to their actions.⁹ A survey of more than four thousand members of the German Society for Internal Medicine (DGIM) shows that measures are carried out or omitted due to financial incentives: 70 percent of the participants state that they are confronted several times a week with the decision whether to perform a measure based on economic considerations.¹⁰ The majority of respondents saw overtreatment as a relevant problem. Overtreatment occurs when medical measures are carried out that have no demonstrable benefit, usually to generate additional revenue.

In the field of oncology, which is quite cost intensive, only a few empirical and interdisciplinary studies on the possible influence of economic factors are available in Germany. A survey of 345 members of the German Society for Hematology and Oncology (DGHO) showed that the respondents fear a deterioration of care as a consequence of cost pressure, and more than half of the participants reported undertreatment—meaning not offering beneficial treatment for cost reasons.¹¹ For cost reasons, 63 percent of the oncologists reported discharging patients prematurely for outpatient care, although inpatient treatment would have made clinical sense. Only a third stated that they had never done so. Sixty-four percent stated that they initially did not use an indicated but expensive measure and waited to see whether the patient could manage without it; fortunately, most of these reported not doing this very often, or less than once

---

7   Giovanni Maio, "Gefährdung der Patientensicherheit im Zeitalter der DRGs," *Zeitschrift für Evidenz Fortbildung und Qualität im Gesundheitswesen* 108, no. 1 (2014): 32–34; and Monika Nothacker et al., "Medizin und Ökonomie: Maßnahmen für eine wissenschaftlich begründete, patientenzentrierte und ressourcenbewusste Versorgung. Ein Strategiepapier der Arbeitsgemeinschaft der Wissenschaftlichen Medizinischen Fachgesellschaften (AWMF)," *Deutsche Medizinische Wochenschrift* 144, no. 14 (2019): 990–96.
8   Deutscher Ethikrat, *Patientenwohl als ethischer Maßstab für das Krankenhaus*, 2016, https://www.ethikrat.org/fileadmin/Publikationen/Stellungnahmen/deutsch/stellungnahme-patientenwohl-als-ethischer-massstab-fuer-das-krankenhaus.pdf.
9   Karl-Heinz Wehkamp and Heinz Naegler, "The Commercialization of Patient-Related Decision Making in Hospitals: A Qualitative Study of the Perceptions of Doctors and Chief Executive Officers," *Deutsches Ärzteblatt International* 114, no. 47 (2017): 797.
10 Gerd Hasenfuß et al., "Initiative 'Klug entscheiden': Gegen Unter- und Überversorgung," *Deutsches Ärzteblatt International* 113, no. 13 (2016): A-600.
11 Stefan W. Krause et al., "Rationing Cancer Care: A Survey among the Members of the German Society of Hematology and Oncology," *Journal of the National Comprehensive Cancer Network* 11, no. 6 (2013): 658–65.

a month. Fifty-nine percent reported that they withheld therapeutic measures for cost reasons, even though the measures were approved and would have a demonstrable advantage over cheaper alternatives, because—in the calculation of these physicians—the therapeutic benefit was too small compared to the difference in cost.[12]

Many oncologists experience a role conflict in making decisions about the provision of indicated but expensive therapies. In particular, the ambivalence between the goal of promoting the well-being of the patient and, at the same time, the need to deal appropriately with the cost pressure on the clinics was viewed as problematic.[13] Hence, many doctors feel caught between two demands—namely, between that of patients, who rightly demand the best available care, and that of society, which expects that physicians, as gatekeepers, must use the system's resources wisely, or even one step further, commercially oriented hospitals, which expect that health care will generate revenue.

Different Strategies to Deal with Cost Pressures and Their Ethical Evaluation

We have seen from reported studies that there are at least three different strategies in practice to respond to cost pressures:
a.) enhancing efficiency to achieve the same result with fewer resources;
b.) increasing revenue—that is, putting more money into the system either by redistributing public money into the health sector or by generating more revenues in the health system itself;
c.) rationing or forgoing effective medical interventions to save money.

In the following, all three strategies are discussed with regard to their ethical justifiability.

Increasing Efficiency

Rationalization, understood as guaranteeing the same treatment result with less resource input, is ethically unproblematic, provided that all relevant input variables are included in the calculation. This excludes, for example, the case where a goal can be achieved only through unpaid overtime or at the expense of time spent talking to patients. In the DRG system, for example, talking medicine in

---

[12] See Hasenfuß et al., "Initiative 'Klug entscheiden.'"
[13] Sandra Fernau et al., "The Role of Physicians in Rationing Cancer Care: Attitudes of German Oncologists," *Oncology Research and Treatment* 40, no. 9 (2017): 490–94.

the sense of involving patients in joint decision-making or involving relatives in the course of treatment is not a basis for remuneration, whereas other services (for example, surgical interventions or ventilation) are constitutive for a DRG case group and thereby a prerequisite for billing. Interdisciplinary or interprofessional coordination is also largely uncompensated. Thus, streamlining this system is likely done at the expense of time for patient-centered care—especially for time- and personnel-intensive treatment of children and adolescents, but also of frail elders. Clarifying complex cases and joint decision-making are therefore not a neutral increase of efficiency.[14]

However, as long as economization in the form of streamlining helps to avoid unnecessary work, cost savings and patient welfare do point in the same direction. This synergism between economy and patient-centeredness can be understood as "good economization." The "Choosing Wisely" initiative aims, for example, at identifying diagnostic and therapeutic interventions for each specialty that can be dispensed without negative consequences for patients.[15] The campaign was initiated in 1989 by the ABIM Foundation (American Board of Internal Medicine) with the goal of advancing the core values of medical professionalism and has spread worldwide, with over eighty medical specialty societies that have published more than six hundred recommendations regarding overused tests and treatments that clinicians and patients should discuss.

Increasing Revenues

One reason for the overuse of medical services is that it generates revenue for the physician's own practice, department, or hospital independent of its medical merits. The above-mentioned survey among members of the German Society of Internal Medicine (DEGIM) illustrates an already existing awareness of the problems related to the negative effects of such an incentive and decision culture: 93 percent of physicians state that health-care expenditures are increased in this way; 63 percent fear that patients are harmed.[16] If health-care services that are not clearly indicated are increasingly offered in order to generate revenue for the physicians' own health-care institution, this represents overuse that cannot be ethically justified, since on one hand such interventions are unnecessarily stressful for patients (and in the worst case even harms them), and on the other hand, such procedures also reduce the available resources for measures that are actually indicated and evidence-based.

---

[14] Deutscher Ethikrat, *Patientenwohl als ethischer Maßstab für das Krankenhaus*.
[15] https://abimfoundation.org/what-we-do/choosing-wisely.
[16] Hasenfuß, "Initiative 'Klug entscheiden.'"

This practice contradicts the oldest medical-ethical commandment, that is, the doctor's obligation to avoid harm *primum non nocere*, and should therefore be rejected from an ethical point of view. It also jeopardizes the medical profession's integrity and patients' trust in the medical profession. On the other hand, the practice does not do justice to society's role as a fair steward of resources if medical interventions are used for unnecessary rather than beneficial measures.

Rationing Health-Care Services

Equally problematic as overtreatment can be undertreatment, when physicians withhold beneficial medical treatments from their patients for cost reasons. This is frequently reported by physicians in Germany (see empirical data above).

Rationing or withholding beneficial treatment is not ethically questionable per se. When it is done explicitly and according to rules agreed upon above the doctor-patient level, then it is even an imperative question that societies must answer: How much are we as a society willing to pay for certain medical innovations and interventions? How many resources should we allocate toward care of children or the elderly, toward programs for prevention or rehabilitation, and so on? Such questions should be addressed in the context of early benefit assessment, before new treatments are approved, and should be informed by principles of public health ethics and discussed by institutions such as the Federal Joint Committee (G-BA) or other deliberative bodies. Many therefore call for an open discussion of the problem and recommend transparent rationing and prioritization according to explicit criteria for the allocation of medical services.

On the doctor-patient level, however, rationing can hardly be justified ethically, because there it works in an implicit, not transparent way—without clear criteria and often without the patient's knowledge. Hence, such action also violates the principles of informed consent, because not all relevant information for a joint decision is passed on to the patient. Implicit rationing also jeopardizes the relationship of trust, since the patient generally assumes that the physician is primarily committed to him or her. Withholding effective measures in individual cases also violates the principle of justice, which is to treat similar cases equally.

The demands made on the physician—the primacy of the patient's well-being, on one hand, and, on the other hand, responsibility for stewardship of society's health-care resources or the financial stability of one's health-care institution—can lead to a conflict of roles.[17] This creates the risk of giving too much

---

[17] Katja Mehlis, Lena Woydack, and Eva C. Winkler, "Klinikkodizes als Korrektiv im ärztlichen Alltag?: Eine Reflexion zur Bedeutungorganisation ethischer Aspekte im Umgang mit der Ökonomisierung des Medizinsystems," *Medizinische Klinik, Intensivmedi-*

weight to economic thinking and putting economic considerations before patient welfare. Giving more weight to economic considerations not only would violate the primary mission of the profession and endanger the quality of care, but also would bring negative consequences for physicians themselves, such as emotional stress, conflicts of conscience, and dishonesty toward the patient if beneficial treatment is withheld.[18]

Normative Approaches and Their Practical Feasibility

Against this background, the German Ethics Council,[19] the Leopoldina,[20] and the AWMF call for a clear "primary orientation" on the welfare of the patient.[21] The analysis so far has shown that the principles of economic action are not necessarily in conflict with an orientation toward patient well-being but may even be required to optimize patient care. On the other hand, it has become clear that in situations where effective therapies are not offered for cost reasons (rationing)—that is, where there is a deviation from the primary orientation toward patient welfare—the level at which these decisions are made is relevant.

Therefore, the focus of this section is on situations in which cost orientation stands in the way of optimal patient care and on the question of which corrective measures are available at the various levels of the health-care system to resolve the tension—with regard to the individual level of medical professionalism, the institutional level of health-care organizations, and the societal and regulatory framework. Especially the institutional level seems to be fruitful in terms of a potential corrective function.

Medical Professionalism as Guidance on the Individual Level

Professional codes of conduct have a long tradition in medicine. They date back to the corpus of the Hippocratic Oath in the fourth century. The oath contains basic ethical expectations that are timeless, such as the principle of nonmaleficence (*primum non nocere*), primary orientation toward the patient's well-being, and the personal integrity of the physician. From the beginning of Western med-

---

zin und Notfallmedizin 115 (2020): https://www.springermedizin.de/klinikkodizes-als-korrektiv-im-aerztlichen-alltag/16715014.

[18] Hasenfuß, "Initiative 'Klug entscheiden.'"
[19] Ibid.
[20] Ibid.
[21] AWMF, "Medizin und Ökonomie—Maßnahmen für eine wissenschaftlich begründete, patientenzentrierte und ressourcenbewusste Versorgung," Mar. 11, 2019.

icine, the question of what makes a good doctor was part of medical training and the self-formation of medicine as a profession. The oath was modernized in 1948 by the World Medical Association as the Geneva Doctors' Pledge—intended to help restore patients' trust in the medical profession after physicians' complicity in Nazi atrocities.[22] The oath is a preamble of the templates of professional regulations of the chambers of physicians in many German-speaking countries since 1956—even if physicians have not regularly pledged to it. More recently, the ceremonial reading of the oath by students graduating from medical school is becoming more and more popular in Germany according to research by *Die Zeit*, and is practiced in seventeen out of thirty-six German medical universities— often at the request of the young doctors.[23] By actually taking an oath, the individual physician realizes the commitment as a member of the profession to its standards. In this way, the oath does not remain a lifeless text but is remembered and forms a professional community committed to the same principles.

In fact, we are currently seeing several movements in this direction. It began with the physician charter of medical professionalism of the professional societies for internal medicine in 2004, which recalls the principles to which the medical profession commits itself in relation to the patient and society.[24] The physician charter sets standards of ethical behavior for physicians and has been endorsed by medical organizations worldwide. It is based on the cardinal principles of the primacy of patient welfare, patient autonomy, and social welfare. These professional codes of conduct are intended to encourage doctors to rely solely on their medical judgment while working primarily for the well-being of patients. The codes are therefore an attempt at self-formation of the profession.[25]

And yet, as we have seen in the first section, the conditions of medical practice in many places are such that the implementation of these principles is coming under increasing pressure. Should the doctor prescribe his patient a cheaper drug with potentially more side effects in order to keep costs down for the general public or the hospital, or should she not offer a treatment with marginal—yet not zero—benefit because it is expensive? These situations often leave the physician feeling morally uneasy and call on the physician's power of judgment to do justice to the individual case and decide on an appropriate course of action.

---

[22] Weltärztebund, "Deklaration von Genf. Das Ärztliche Gelöbnis," https://www.bundesaerztekammer.de/fileadmin/user_upload/BAEK/Themen/Internationales/Bundesaerztekammer_Deklaration_von_Genf_04.pdf.

[23] Harro Albrecht, "Zeit für einen neuen Eid," *Die Zeit*, Nov. 12, 2015, p 46.

[24] AWMF, "Medizin und Ökonomie."

[25] Eva C. Winkler, "Verwirklichung des ärztlichen Ethos—Die Selbstformung von Ärzten," in *Selbstformung—Beiträge zur Aufklärung einer menschlichen Praxis*, ed. Ruth Congrad and Roland Kipke (Münster: Mentis Verlag, 2015), 241–57.

More generally, which conditions enable ethical decision-making in the clinic? In what follows I would like to show that the conditions for ethically defensible solutions in difficult decision-making situations in the clinic are to be found both at the individual doctor-patient level and in the institutional embeddedness and framework. Practical judgment and institutional ethics reinforce each other.

Expectations toward Organizational Ethics

Clinical ethics is primarily concerned with moral questions with a focus on the individual doctor-patient relationship. In recent years, however, it has been emphasized more and more strongly that value-based decisions do not take place in a vacuum but are instead embedded in institutional contexts—even more than that, in the context of complex organizations, such as hospitals. Thus, if the economic framework is experienced as ethically problematic, in tension, or even incompatible with medical professional values, an ethical corrective function at a higher level is necessary. This level is addressed by so-called organizational ethics. Organizational ethics can be understood as ethics within the organization and as "inter" ethics between macro and micro ethics, and thus includes ethical behavior within the organization—for example, by defining ethical standards and ethical behavior of employees—as well as ethical behavior of the organization itself. The sociology of organizations theory about people acting in complex organizations provides helpful insights here.[26] Organizational structures and incentives influence, but do not determine, the motivation and decision of the individuals who are socialized into a certain organizational culture and exposed to a specific organizational climate. A theory of institutional ethics should therefore do justice to the decision of the acting individual, the structures in which this action is embedded, and the mutual influence of the two.[27] Hence, as a theory, organizational ethics analyzes (a) the principles that guide decisions and responsible behavior and (b) the conditions that the institution should create for its employees to act ethically.[28] As practice, organizational ethics includes the

---

[26] Anthony Giddens, *The Constitution of Society: Outline of the Theory of Structuration* (Cambridge: Polity Press, 1984).

[27] Eva C. Winkler, "The Ethics of Policy Writing: How Should Hospitals Deal with Moral Disagreement about Controversial Medical Practices?," *Journal of Medical Ethics* 31 (2005): 559–66.

[28] Eva C. Winkler and Russell L. Gruen, "First Principles: Substantive Ethics for Healthcare Organizations," *Journal of Healthcare Management* 50, no. 2 (2005):109–19; discussion 119–20.

establishment of processes that ensure that the institution lives up to its responsibility to all stakeholders.[29]

Empirical studies on factors influencing value-based behavior in an organization show that morally correct behavior is promoted in an organization if the leadership provides a clear guideline in the sense of a code of conduct and, within the framework of this, rewards ethically responsible behavior while sanctioning negative behavior.[30] Such factors contribute to the corporate culture and ethical climate of an organization and have a systematic influence on the handling of value-laden situations. While this theory is certainly applicable to health-care institutions, it is important to emphasize the responsibility of each individual physician to live up to the professional ideal of the primacy of the patient's good. If this ideal builds the basis of a code of conduct for the entire institution and guides institutional policies on resource allocation, it can be very powerful. However, the implementation of such a code or policy is not a trivial last step in the deliberative process; it is the very essence of taking seriously what we know about organizations. It is the point at which research in organizational theory, learning behavior, and culture is brought to bear.

Senior leadership, especially in hierarchical organizations, must enthrone the code in order to add the "status authority" to the "competence authority" it should already possess. One example for such a code is the Clinic Code of the German Society for Internal Medicine (DEGIM).[31] The code emphasizes the primacy of the patient's well-being over financial obligations and thus reacts directly to the profit orientation or bad version of economization of the medical system. Physicians should thus be offered a basis for argumentation, so that their medical actions are always geared toward the well-being of the patient.

This voluntary commitment of health-care professionals is written in the first person plural—"we." (The Hippocratic Oath and the Geneva Pledge are written in the first person singular.) Effects of economization on medical patient relationship and therapy decisions are reflected in this context: "As a medical profession, we are committed to using our available resources as efficiently and economically as possible. At the same time, we always focus on the well-being of our patients."[32] While this code could be a powerful tool of institutional ethics, it is formulated only for the medical profession and puts physicians somewhat in opposition to the management, and maybe unrightfully so. Extending core val-

---

[29] Eva C. Winkler, "Organisatorische Ethik—ein erweiterter Auftrag für klinische Ethikkomitees?," in *Wie viel Ethik verträgt die Medizin*, ed. Marcus Düwell and Josef N. Neumann (Paderborn: Mentis, 2005).

[30] Hasenfuß, "Initiative 'Klug entscheiden.'"

[31] Petra-Maria Schumm-Draeger et al., " Ökonomisierung in der Medizin, Rückhalt für ärztliches Handeln," *Deutsches Ärzteblatt* 114, no. 49 (2017): A2338–40.

[32] Ibid, A2340.

ues to all representatives of the leadership, including the management and hospital administration, is an essential step for supporting incentives that foster the best patient outcomes and abandon those that jeopardize them.

Conclusion

Physicians see themselves as increasingly influenced by economic considerations in their actions, and empirical data show that cost pressures impact medical care. This can have positive effects in terms of increased efficiency, but certainly also a negative impact on the doctor-patient relationship and the quality of treatment. A reflection on an appropriate form of economization in the medical system therefore seems necessary. While economic considerations are to be welcomed if they increase efficiency and avoid unnecessary services in the health-care system, overtreatment for financial gains is ethically not permissible, and rationing is so only if it is done explicitly and above the doctor-patient level.

The normative guidelines that define the corridor of medical action are grounded in professional ethics (medical professionalism) and organizational ethics of health-care institutions.[33] Medical professionalism commits physicians to the cardinal principles of the primacy of patient welfare, patient autonomy, and social welfare, and encourages physicians in their aim of working primarily for the well-being of their patients. Pledges to these professional principles, codes, and oaths are one way of nurturing professional self-assurance and expressing the seriousness of self-commitment. However, when these principles cannot be implemented in practice and are countered by stronger (economic) forces, such codes and oaths tend to be a source of frustration. In the end, what is needed is a commitment by all leadership of the health-care system to patient well-being while spending resources reasonably—especially by all hospital leadership of health-care organizations. The principles for such a leadership have been laid out in terms of organizational ethics for health-care organizations. Organizational ethics thus enables all health-care professionals and hospital leadership to live up to the professional ethical principles to which they are committed.

---

[33] Winkler and Gruen, "First Principles: Substantive Ethics for Healthcare Organizations."

Mercy under Conditions of Scarcity and the Need for Organization; or, Where Is the Humane Ethos Located in the Health-Care System? An Outline of the Problem

Günter Thomas

The following theses outline an analysis of the social distribution of values in the system of health care and address the resulting conflicts. A special focus is on the relationship of diverging value orientations in the organizational form of the health-care system. In order to understand the presence of value conflicts in hospitals, it is necessary to consider the so-called cultural-religious antecedents.

The Theological-Historical Background

An ethos of caring for the sick is deeply inscribed in Christianity. It is rooted, among other things, in Jesus's healings of the sick, which in turn are to be seen in the trajectory of divine attention to bodily life in the incarnation. The healings of the sick are an integral part of Jesus's actions, occurring in all the Gospels, albeit with different theological emphases. They include a caring attention to damaged life, regardless of the expected "efficiency" and value of the sick people. In other words, the healings of the sick thematize unacceptable risks of creaturely bodily life and therefore shape a religious-human ethos.

By the end of the fifth century, three outcomes had emerged from Jesus's healings in terms of healing the sick and the ethos of mercy:

(a) The metaphorizing tradition of *Christus medicus*—which took medicine as the guiding model for the theological imagination and construction of the spiritual life—was powerful in antiquity and can be found in therapeutic forms of thought in theology up to the present.[1]

---

[1] Jörg Hübner, "Christus medicus: ein Symbol des Erlösungsgeschehens und ein Modell ärztlichen Handelns," *Kerygma und Dogma* 31 (1985): 324–35; Martin Honecker, "Christus medicus," *Kerygma und Dogma* 31 (1985): 307–23; and, especially, Michael Dörnemann, "Einer ist Arzt, Christus. Krankheitsdeutung in den Schriften der frühen griechischen Kirchenväter," in *Krankheitsdeutung in der postsäkularen Gesellschaft. The-*

b) The tradition of healing miracles, which were later associated with special persons (saints) or special spiritual presences. This tradition maintained, and continues to maintain, a close relationship with the supernatural, the extraordinary miracle, and the spiritual gift of special healers.[2]

c) In the shadow of these first two traditions, the tradition of classical care of the sick developed early in the context of the prevailing medicine.[3] With this attention to the sick corresponded very early a disproportionate share of Christians among physicians, measured by the share of Christians in the population.[4]

In the second or third generation after the building of a church, at the latest, Christian communities established infirmaries. They were partly financed by foundations and always open to nonmembers of the congregations. At least for the churches of the West, it is undeniable that a distinctive value structure fostered a system of care for the sick. In conjunction with this value orientation, supported by technical innovation and scientific research, the modern Western health-care system emerged.

The Problem

Even in the present, the formulation of values, preferences, and moral impositions is almost universally carried out in models of thought oriented toward the personal I-Thou encounter. This orientation overlooks the fact that, in late modern societies, most of the common life beyond family interaction takes place in organizations. This is especially true of the health-care system.[5]

---

ologische Ansätze im interdisziplinären Gespräch, ed. Günter Thomas and Isolde Karle (Stuttgart: Kohlhammer, 2009), 247–60; and Michael Dörnemann, *Krankheit und Heilung in der Theologie der frühen Kirchenväter* (Tübingen: Mohr Siebeck, 2003).

[2] For a more recent appropriation of this tradition, see Jan-Olav Henriksen and Karl Olav Sandnes, *Jesus as Healer: A Gospel for the Body* (Grand Rapids: Eerdmans, 2016).

[3] Gary B. Ferngren, "Krankheit," in *Reallexikon für Antike und Christentum*, ed. Theodore Klauser (Stuttgart: Anton Hiersemann Verlag, 2006), 21:966–1006; Otto Hiltbrunner, "Krankenhaus," in Klauser, *Reallexikon für Antike und Christentum*, 21:882–914; Manfred Wacht, "Krankenfürsorge," in Klauser, *Reallexikon für Antike und Christentum*, 21:826–82; and Gary B. Ferngren, *Medicine and Health Care in Early Christianity* (Baltimore: Johns Hopkins University Press, 2009).

[4] Christian Schulze, *Medizin und Christentum in Spätantike und frühem Mittelalter. Christliche Ärzte und ihr Wirken* (Tübingen: Mohr Siebeck, 2005); and Christian Schulze and Sibylle Ihm, eds., *Ärztekunst und Gottvertrauen. Antike und mittelalterliche Schnittpunkte von Christentum und Medizin* (Hildesheim: G. Olms Verlag, 2002).

[5] On the systemic nature of medical organizations and communications, see Werner Vogd, "Medizinsystem und Gesundheitswissenschaften—Rekonstruktion einer schwieri-

The question must therefore be asked, where and at what points in complex organizations striving for effectiveness do values in fact determine health care. The issue is the social distribution of values in health-care organizations, which are undoubtedly not always free of conflict.[6] When a health-care system is to be transformed or optimized and developed in the face of new challenges, this distribution of values affects these systemic switches in their entirety. Tensions within the organizations of the health-care system are mostly tensions between the value orientations of natural as well as institutional actors—because not only natural persons but also nonnatural persons realize value preferences.

The Current Constellation in the Health-Care System

The Organization

Organizations ultimately consist of decisions.[7] They lead to the establishment of formative structures and initiate, but also maintain, procedures and processes. The value preferences of the organization may well differ from the value pref-

---

gen Beziehung," *Soziale Systeme* 11 (2005): 236–70; Werner Vogd, "Kontexturen der Heilung in einer polykontexturalen Gesellschaft. Empirische und gesellschaftstheoretische Untersuchungen zur Koexsitenz scheinbar widersprüchlicher Semantiken," in Thomas and Karle, *Krankheitsdeutung in der postsäkularen Gesellschaft*, 23–35; and Gunnar Stollberg, "Das medizinische System. Überlegungen zu einem von der Soziologie vernachlässigten Funktionssystem," *Soziale Systeme* 15 (2009): 189–217.

[6] On value conflict, see the excellent study by Ulrich Willems, *Wertkonflikte als Herausforderung der Demokratie* (Wiesbaden: Springer, 2016), who clearly differentiates conflicts of interest and value conflicts. For value conflicts in organizational settings, see, among others, Christiane Staffhorst, *Wertkonflikte in Unternehmen Eine erweiterte organisationstheoretische Analyse von Korruption* (Wiesbaden: Springer, 2010); elaborating value conflicts in medicine, yet without taking the organizational issues into account, see Hartmut Kreb, *Medizinische Ethik: Gesundheitsschutz, Selbstbestimmungsrechte, heutige Wertkonflikte* (Stuttgart: Kohlhammer, 2009). After almost fifty years, still illuminating is Laurence H. Tribe et al., eds., *When Values Conflict: Essays on Environmental Analysis, Discourse, and Decision* (Cambridge, Mass.: Ballinger,1976). In a very fundamental way remaining skeptical about the guiding role of values, Niklas Luhmann, "Die Moral des Risikos und das Risiko der Moral," in id., *Risiko und Gesellschaft: Grundlagen und Ergebnisse interdiziplinärer Risikoforschung*, ed. Gotthard Bechmann (Wiesbaden: Verlag für Sozialwissenschaften, 1993), 327–38; and Niklas Luhmann, *Die Moral der Gesellschaft* (Frankfurt am Main: Suhrkamp, 2008).

[7] Niklas Luhmann, *Organisation und Entscheidung* (Wiesbaden: VS Verlag, 2000); and Niklas Luhmann, "Lob der Routine," in *Politische Planung* (Opladen: Westdeutscher Verlag, 1971), 113–42.

erences of the medical staff or even the patients. It is true, however, that organizations, and thus hospitals, rely on boundary setting and selectivity in environmental sensitivity. Inclusion in the organization—that is, the treatment of patients—cannot be boundaryless and can only ever be "discriminating" and, thus, boundary setting. Complex and costly organizations, such as health-care organizations, can be "merciful" only within narrow limits and can act beyond rights and obligations as well as beyond their internal logic.

The problem of limitation also occurs in the core of the organization. All organizations that not only provide the solution to a problem, but also are instrumental in discovering and identifying the underlying problem to be solved, are tempted to discover more and more of their own underlying problem. Thus, an additional problem reveals itself, namely, that problem identification can get so out of hand that, in principle, there can and must be "even more" problem solving. This inflationary expansion can be observed in many places in medicine, religion, pedagogy, economics, and, not least, in law. Attempts to counteract it are manifold.

Funding

Organizations in particular need a certainty of expectation in financing, which is why they prefer organizations in financing—specifically, insurance companies. In the Federal Republic of Germany, health-insurance companies, as independent actors, do not necessarily represent the interests of other organizations—that is, medical practices and hospitals. Depending on state-specific regulations, health insurers pursue their own financial agenda, but help determine what can be done in hospitals. The interests and values of the various organizations in the health-care system need not coincide. What is indisputable, however, is that for all the supposed boundlessness of humanity, love, and a human rights ethos based on solidarity, the financial possibilities of any health-care organization are limited.

The Financiers

Public or government funding of health care requires the approval of voters. Voters must be willing to contribute money to a community of solidarity, for example, through insurance premiums or public budgets. Voters thus ultimately regulate the exclusion and inclusion of potential patients in the health-care system. An international comparison shows how unlikely and preconditioned a public health-care system with corresponding medical services is. A look at the United States shows that even a high degree of religiosity does not necessarily lead quickly to such communities of solidarity that support the health-care system and are socially far-reaching. Increased individual compassion and willingness to help may be accompanied by a reluctance to form national and, in complex ways, organizational communities of solidarity.

Human Actors and Clinical Staff

Organizations are not made up of people, but they operate largely in the medium of people. Thus, medical personnel are part of the hospital only in a very specific sense. Nevertheless, nurses and physicians always interpret and vary the rules of the organization in multiple ways: "duty by the book" can be interpreted as sabotage. This consideration makes it clear that physicians and nurses bring their own ethos and values to the framework of the hospital organization. One could speak of a moral style or a value style with which they give life to the spaces of the organization, which are in part morally overdetermined and in part morally underdetermined.

Patients

Against the background of the rules of the organization, the financing of the organization, and the legal regulations, potential and real patients (including their relatives) develop very specific expectations of the organization and the medical staff. In these expectations toward the health-care organization and its representatives, value attitudes are realized at the same time.

The Challenges

It would be surprising, indeed downright naïve, to assume a complete fit of multiple value preferences. In my opinion, however, it would also be insufficiently complex to try to identify primarily value conflicts. Without assuming a complete fit and without assuming a war of value orientations in the organizations of the health-care system, it is a matter of specifically recognizing value conflicts as well as mutual reinforcements in the value orientations.

It is undisputed that for a well-functioning health-care system, corresponding positive value preferences preserving the function of the organization are necessary among all actors: excessive patient expectations can "lead the medical system to the brink" just as much as inadequate funding, just as much as an organization working with the wrong goals, or even medical staff without an ethos. The first challenge, then, is to sensibly orchestrate the various value systems or value orientations and the associated expectations. Against the background of this complex constellation, unilateral appeals to the values of, for example, medical staff will come to nothing so long as the organization sets inappropriate framework conditions.

Another challenge is that the various actors in the health-care organization also observe each other's value orientations. The results of this observation are fed into the actors' own future options for action. One option for action, but not the only one, that results from this mutual observation is the consideration of the values of others for the assertion of one's own interests and value orientations. For example, when medical staff get into "orientational distress," it is usually because the organization considers the ethos of the staff in its structures and processes, but economizes for efficiency and cost-saving goals in the very process. In this case, the health-care organization does not care about the health of its staff. After all, according to the operationally effective insinuation, fewer people with a high ethos can do the same work. Because of these observational operations, an ethos that focuses solely on the compassion of hospital staff leads to destructive forms of self-exploitation by the staff. Hospital organizations, however, may also observe the preferences of health insurers and develop their own preferences contrary to insurer expectations. Through observations, value preferences evolve into cleverness calculi.

Another challenge is that value orientations are arguably too weak to limit expectation inflation. This concerns the expectations of patients and relatives about the services of medical practices and hospitals, but also the expectations imposed by health insurers on hospitals and, last but not least, the expectations imposed by organizations on their employees (the DRG system in Germany is an attempt to regulate this diversity of expectations). What can, what must, and what may the health-care system provide? What may patients rightfully expect from physicians, what may physicians expect from nurses, what may economic management expect from physicians, what may physicians expect from patients, etc.? What role do deeply rooted cultural values play in the cultivation and inflation of expectations, but also in the limitation of claims (the ethos of self-restraint and renunciation)—without this being immediately exploited in turn by the observation operations of other actors? To put it in classical terms of ethical theory, how do value preferences operate in regulating the rights and duties of different actors?

As much as Christianity is able to emphasize the boundlessness of love, it is structurally necessary and indispensable to draw boundaries within organizations and vis-à-vis their environments. Organized communities of solidarity must always be inclusive and exclusive at the same time in order to function effectively. Without state boundaries—that is, without the distinction between civil rights and human rights—it is not possible to build a system of state solidarity assistance with many organizations. (This includes a sense of we, a cultural identity, a cultural community of trust—in short, a nation). The inherent tragedy of limitation must be recognized and must not be covered up with moral maximum demands. This also applies to the organizations of the health-care system. If health-care systems are organized and financed through a community of solidarity, they can include sick people only at the price of exclusion.[8]

If one looks at the health-care systems in an international comparison, one sees how a decisive question is answered differently in many different ways. The question that has to be answered in different ways then also concerns the training of guiding preferences and the hierarchization of values. The question is, to which social system do hospitals and medical centers belong? From the point of view of systems theory, in all social subsystems, the organizations concerned are the places where the services of other systems are used. In courts, for instances, bailiffs are paid, art is hung, and press releases are written without the right becoming a commodity. Correspondingly, in health-care organizations, the services of law, religion, media, education, and science are always claimed as well. Nevertheless, the social subsystems—Max Weber spoke of spheres of value—differ strikingly in their guiding orientation. The legal system may pay its judges, but it does not sell law.

And yet there seems to be an internal tipping point in the question of financing health-care organizations. Apparently, in some countries, health care is assigned to the economic system. Hospitals then sell health-care services directly to solvent customers in an attempt to make a profit.[9] This is then done without the regulative idea of a common good.

Conversely, there are also attempts to assign health-care organizations ultimately to the religious system. The entrepreneurial Diakonie in Germany sees itself as a "witness to the gospel" and claims to follow its own "third way" in employment relationships as well—without being able to escape economic constraints and dynamics and without being able to act on the basis of lavish love and truly boundless mercy.[10] Whether it makes sense to speak of hybrid orga-

---

[8] On the dialectics of inclusion and exclusion, see Armin Nassehi, "Die paradoxe Einheit von Inklusion und Exklusion. Ein systemtheoretischer Blick auf die 'Phänomene,'" in *Das Problem der Exklusion. Ausgegrenzte, Entbehrliche, Überflüssige*, ed. Heinz Bude and Andreas Willisch (Hamburg: Hamburger Edition, 2006), 46–69.

[9] The issue of economization is part and parcel of all debates about the U.S. health care system.

[10] See the constitution of the Union of Protestant Churches, Article 15: "Die Evangelische Kirche in Deutschland und die Gliedkirchen sind gerufen, Christi Liebe in Wort und Tat zu verkündigen. 2 Diese Liebe verpflichtet alle Glieder der Kirche zum Dienst und gewinnt in besonderer Weise Gestalt im Diakonat der Kirche; demgemäß sind die diakonisch-missionarischen Werke Wesens- und Lebensäußerung der Kirche." [(1) The Evangelical Church in Germany and the member churches are called to proclaim Christ's

nizations in these cases is an open question that needs to be clarified. The fact is, however, that diaconal organizations in the health-care system openly advertise their Christian value preferences and value hierarchies.

In the context of organizations in the health-care system, a problem arises that is hardly dealt with in theological and philosophical ethics, but which is nevertheless pressing: which value orientations should or must be transferred from the realm of personal ethos into legal regulations? Which should deliberately not? Particularly organizations that work quickly under time pressure, and in which many people have to work together, need a high degree of certainty of expectations, which is established either by voluntary, ethically enforced and time-binding routines or by explicit sets of rules. The side effect is then a density of rules that grows with the problem stories, making the space of individual responsibility almost disappear. At the same time, however, the separation of legality (compliance with rules) and morality (justification by personal ethos) relieves the burden.

Concluding Considerations on Orientational Distress

In the whole arrangement of a modern health-care system, it is not only the case that value orientations are present and functional orientations are effective on the part of all actors. Rather, broader visions of a good, fulfilled, and successful life are also built in—always depending on medially, religiously, or politically grounded conceptions of the good and just life. Because these visions are deeply embedded and often represent blind spots, it seems questionable whether they can be directly addressed, discussed, critiqued, and reshaped. Lifting the truly effective, integrating, and more comprehensive values out of their so-called latent protection always makes them appear riskily contingent as well. On the other hand, the formation of health-care organizations should not be left to markets and short-term political cycles alone. Churches and, by extension, religious communities can be places where the latently effective visions of a good life can be discussed—without damaging the latent protection in the health-care organization itself.

It is in the medical personnel where the tensions and conflicts of the value orientations of the entire organization play out. These tensions can be resolved only if nurses and physicians have a high degree of moral navigational skills

---

love in word and deed. 2 This love commits all members of the church to service and takes special shape in the diaconate of the church; accordingly, diaconal and missionary organizations are an essential and vital expression of the church.]: https://www.kirchenrecht-ekd.de/document/3435#s1.100023. To frame the issue in another way: There is an unsolvable tension between mercy and justice.

amid conflicting expectations and value orientations. This became abundantly clear during the Covid pandemic. The pandemic brought medical personnel worldwide to the brink of exhaustion.[11] It carried more than a few physicians and nurses beyond that. In the process, the pandemic brought home forcefully the problem of orientational distress.[12]

Medical professions can indeed experience what can be called orientational distress.[13] This is a situation of breakdown in the patterns of orientational self-understanding on which nurses and physicians normally rely. Routine expectations, decision-making procedures, and common-sense relationships between professional and personal life are turned upside down in such a way that the well-being of both the individual and the institution is threatened. The ability to navigate within and amidst divergent value orientations is lost. Typical support tools used to address this loss—such as coaching, psychotherapy, and yoga—are often insufficient to solve the problem.[14] These approaches focus on the individual professional and precisely not on the organization with its specific challenges and dynamics.

Orientational distress as a loss of navigational ability and paralyzing value orientation conflict always occurs in the interactions between institutions and their employees. Religiously based value orientations are likely to prove highly ambivalent in the situation of orientational distress. On one hand, the spiritual-theological grounding promotes an irritation resistance of value orientations and thus, psychologically, increases a value resilience. On the other hand, in corrosive environments with exploitative value observations of others and corre-

---

[11] See, for example, M. Luo et al., "The Psychological and Mental Impact of Coronavirus Disease 2019 (COVID-19) on Medical Staff and General Public–A Systematic Review and Meta-Analysis," *Psychiatry* Research 291 (2020): 113190; and Y. K. Song et al., "Morally Injurious Experiences and Emotions of Health Care Professionals during the COVID-19 Pandemic before Vaccine Availability," *JAMA Netw Open* 4 (2021): e2136150; and M. Denning et al., "Determinants of Burnout and Other Aspects of Psychological Well-Being in Healthcare Workers during the Covid-19 Pandemic: A Multinational Cross-Sectional Study," *PLoS One* 16 (2021), e0238666.

[12] For a more detailed elaboration of the concept of orientational distress see Günter Thomas et al., *The Enhancing Life Laboratory: Tools for Addressing Orientational Distress in the Medical Profession Academic Medicine* (under review) (2023).

[13] Orientational distress is a broader concept than moral distress, since it has components of cognitive orientation. For moral distress, see Diya Banerjee and Yesne Alici, "Moral Distress in Physicians," in *Depression, Burnout and Suicide in Physicians: Insights from Oncology and other Medical Professions*, ed. Luigi Grassi et al. (Cham: Springer, 2022), 127–35.

[14] S. Mantri et al., "Reframing the Conversation around Physician Burnout and Moral Injury: 'We're Not Suffering From a Yoga Deficiency,'" *Permanente Journal* 25 (2021), https://www.ncbi.nlm.nih.gov/pmc/articles/PMC8784069/.

sponding hot value conflicts, the irritation-resilience of moral commitment can also lead to deep exhaustion under conditions of intensified finitude. Whenever this happens, there can be a continuum between orientational distress and eventually burnout.[15] Especially a Protestant theology and piety will at this point hold an ultimate relativity of all moral endeavors as liberating gospel.

---

[15] The intimate connection between high values and burnout is highlighted by the most recent detailed study by George Mayzell, *The Resilient Healthcare Organization: How to Reduce Physician and Healthcare Worker Burnout* (New York: Productivity Press, 2020), as well as National Academies of Sciences, Engineering, and Medicine, *Taking Action against Clinician Burnout: A Systems Approach to Professional Well-Being* (Washington, DC: National Academies Press, 2019).

Ethical Tensions in the Medical Treatment of Elderly Patients in Geriatrics and Geriatric Psychiatry

Christine Thomas

The medical care of elderly patients is first of all characterized by a long life history and the associated manifold experiences of the subjective perception of illness and health, as well as confrontation with objectively diagnosed—though often denied—chronic diseases. Experiences of one's own and other people's phases of illness, care situations, and the company of close relatives in illnesses over the entire life span into aging and finally into a timely or untimely death all bear the potential for conflict over a patient's sovereignty of interpretation and decision-making, both between the generations and between medical and therapeutic practitioners. Fears of lost status and autonomy because of chronic illness, disability, or neurodegenerative diseases, such as Parkinson's disease or dementia, often hinder unconditional openness to consultation and care. Differences in objective assessments and subjective perceptions of resources and competencies often result in (unrealistic) concerns about the excessive care burden on close relatives or the financial strain of nursing home costs and other related expenses. The interests of patients themselves often differ from those of their relatives or following generations.

In caring for the elderly and people with chronic disabilities, tensions arise from the interplay of their self-esteem with the role they or others ascribe to them in the family, the quality of life the patients themselves perceive, and their attitudes toward therapy risks, therapy limitation, containment of suffering, and even a self-determined end of life.

Demographic developments, with further increases in life expectancy, are leading to a rise in the number of old and very old patients. At the same time, modern medicine, with minimally invasive procedures, secondary prevention, and broad diagnostics, has come a long way in developing treatment of older patients. Patients over the age of sixty-five make up the majority of hospital patients. However, the increase in "healthy years" also leads to increasing economic pressure on hospitals, health-insurance companies, and outpatient and inpatient care providers, as well as on the entire health-care system and society.

Ethical conflicts and dilemmas arise here on at least three levels. First, at the level of the patient, who is supposed to make autonomously informed decisions through living wills and participatory decision-making requirements. Conflicts arise here because of the interpretative leeway of many living wills. In particular, the "deselection" of certain forms of treatment (for example, artificial nutrition or ventilation) sometimes does not anticipate the need for medical monitoring of electrolyte imbalances to avoid potentially fatal cardiac arrhythmias, or for bridging of independent nutrition in the case of swallowing disorders or delirium (acute confusion) caused by a lack of fluids. Often there is only a reference to an advance directive as a document limiting therapy, without the actual regulations being perceived and known.

To prevent patients' wishes from being misinterpreted and their quality of life and prospects for therapy from being misjudged, the practice of ethics discussions has become established in hospitals and nursing homes. This practice brings together attending physicians from various disciplines, nursing staff from the intensive and long-term care areas, social workers, relatives or friends, as well as pastoral counselors, and, if possible, even the patient to weigh the various options under professional moderation (an ethics adviser) and consider the presumed best therapy and life options. In most cases, the principles of utilitarian ethics are applied; individual partial interests are named and evaluated accordingly. For example, the decision to temporarily administer fluids may become possible if the procedure can enhance the quality of life in the short term, or a palliative situation may be reevaluated under the expert psychiatric assessment of a treatable depression. In addition, the severity of the need for care and the resulting burden on partners, children, and relatives can sometimes be assessed differently than was possible by the patient alone.

On the other hand, physicians' rejections of unrealistic demands for maximum therapy become more understandable through the specialist's detailed explanation of the objective lack of efficacy of, for example, resuscitation measures in old age or with regard to the physical strain of days of ventilation in the case of severe pneumonia, given the background of already advanced frailty or cognitive impairment.

Rescue services and emergency physicians, however, often find themselves in situations where information is lacking or wrong, and they then depend on verbal statements from individuals present—for example, in the nursing home. This often results in overprovision of care in an emergency situation due to lack of documentation of a therapeutic focus strictly oriented to quality of life, leading in turn to misallocated economic resources and a seemingly inhumane action.

At the same time, a nihilism in the treatment of very old people arising from the personal misjudgment of quality of life in illness and disability must be resisted. Such nihilism prevents a thorough consideration of the life situation and bears the risk that therapeutic actions are omitted which could alleviate suffering, or that the patient's autonomy is unduly restricted.

For example, mobility is an important expression of autonomy, especially in the face of increasingly limited cognitive resources. The ability to walk, especially in a nursing home, can enable independent choice about where to engage in the community or whether to retreat into the private sphere in everyday life, and should therefore be maintained or promoted as long as possible. This autonomy must then also be weighed against a risk of falling or self-endangerment due to orientation disorders. The claim on behalf of the greatest possible safety of the patient, which is demanded by relatives but also by health-insurance companies and home supervision, is often mistaken here, since it unduly limits the decisions of the patient's natural and free will.

On the other hand, a laissez-faire attitude must be contradicted, because it overemphasizes a purely fateful course and often withdraws the assumption of responsibility and the need for caring decision-making. Accommodation of a patient in a protected area for those experiencing dementia, while leaving them the possibility of protected access to a garden, for example, ultimately allows more autonomy and quality of life than the medicinal prevention of active participation in everyday life through sedation and inhibition of movement.

However, dilemmas also arise when patients for many years have avoided dealing with the impositions of physiological aging and age-associated diseases, so that further intrapsychic development can no longer take place. One-sidedly formed couple relationships can also lead to excessive demands, and superhuman expectations of care services by relatives or financial dependencies can be the basis for maintaining a status quo that is ultimately detrimental to quality of life. Unrealistic hopes for medical success or stubborn adherence to a living situation that ultimately represents a gilded cage and prevents everyday satisfaction often require careful guidance and education of medical and nursing professionals.

Here, however, it is also necessary to look at the current possibilities of the actors in the health-care system, who are often burdened with immense time pressure and economic coercion from health-insurance companies and facility operators. This situation presents a special challenge to make time for clarifying discussions and complex decision-making while including, for example, a hearing-impaired patient or overprotective, partially dependent relatives. In the fast-paced daily hospital routine, it is often difficult to allow sufficient time for the process of arriving at such jointly supported decisions.

Bed shortages, the lack of adequate home structures, and the unwillingness of patients and relatives to accept change are obstacles here. The refusal of the social and health-care system to provide sufficient resources for necessary investments in structures and buildings, to provide transitional arrangements (for example, sufficient short-term and interim care options), or to enable appropriate adjustments to the medical infrastructure (for example, adapting hospital structures to the needs of the elderly and cognitively impaired), and the attitude of society as a whole of a postulated loss of quality of life in the case of physical and cognitive impairments—all of these factors promote the overvaluation of a pseudo-autonomous (because ultimately fear-driven) decision to a self-determined end of life, which is then classified as "more dignified." Regulatory failures to provide adapted living space and to take over care for those in need at the borders of society (addicts, the homeless, those who are difficult to integrate socially, and people who do not seek help, for instance) must be corrected.

In addition, the deficits in hospital financing, especially in medical care for the old and the oldest-old stand in stark contrast to medical advances in diagnostics and therapy, the general increase in costs, and the growing, unrealistic expectations of relatives and patients, which are partly influenced by society, the media, and even health-insurance funds. Hospital costs represent the largest area of expenditure for health-insurance funds. The claim to "sufficient, appropriate, but not exceeding the necessary quality of treatment"[1] anchored in the social laws of Germany is not communicated in this way to the individual health-insurance policyholder, who expects high-quality, patient-centered care with the best possible end result. This performance requirement also contrasts with the orientation toward patient welfare as an ethical standard called for by the German Ethics Council in its statement of April 2016.[2] This discrepancy between the reality of the profession and the professional ethos ultimately leads to the exploitation of the good will and ideals of medical and nursing staff and to their frequently leaving the profession—or leaving it emotionally and mentally, and thus turning away from their vocation.

In contrast, society should rather be confronted with the demand to provide humane companionship and professional care until death and to provide education about the possibilities of pain- and suffering-free abstention from food and fluids at the end of life. Particularly in the case of dementia, which is ultimately fatal, it is especially important to use quality of life as a guideline in order not to either underprovide or overprovide care, not to inappropriately limit autonomy or inappropriately reject care. At the same time, however, the demand on society and the individual must be formulated to do justice to this ethical responsibility, to distribute resources fairly and honor the willingness to finance the security systems as a community of solidarity, to ward off abuse, and to anchor both care and security in law.

In addition, a return to the principle of no harm, or *nil nocere*, must be demanded in medical practice. This professional orientation toward evidence-

---

[1] Social Code (SGB) Book Five (V)—Statutory Health Insurance, Section 39.
[2] The German Ethics Council: "The Well-Being of Patients as an Ethical Benchmark for Hospitals." Official Statement. German Ethics Council, Berlin, 2016.

based guidelines—which, however, always uses scientific findings on cohorts with ideal conditions as a basis and has not examined multimorbid and aging people in particular—must therefore be supplemented by experience and empathy for the life situation of the individual. Initiatives such as "Choosing Wisely" in the United States, which fights overmedication, and the "Klug entscheiden!" (Decide wisely!) initiative of the German Society of Internal Medicine, which ultimately focuses on underuse and overmedication of the individual patient as a quality initiative, are positive developments.

The current burdens on service providers ultimately damage professional ethics in the long term because of covert rationing without clear normative guidelines, a situation that enormously impairs the doctor-patient relationship and significantly reduces job satisfaction. In contrast, targeted face-to-face communication between treatment providers and patients can be a resource to optimally support individual value decisions with good professional advice. In this way, a patient's wishes can be validly formed and recorded, and, at the same time, a competence can be developed in dealing with putting them in writing, which can represent a reflected guideline for medical and nursing actions. Remaining conflicts and dilemmas can be resolved or minimized in interdisciplinary and interprofessional communication with patients and relatives—if necessary, under the moderation of an ethics adviser.

Part Two: Ethical Impacts of Advancing Medical Research and Techniques

The Impact of Advances in Stem Cell and Genome Research on Ethical Decision-Making

Anthony D. Ho

As a hematologist/oncologist with special focus on stem cell transplant and stem cell research for over thirty years, I have been exposed to the medical and health care systems in Germany, the United Kingdom, Canada, the United States, and finally back in Germany again. I am pleased to share with you a few stories. The first are stories of two of my patients in their respective battles against cancer, followed by the story of the convoluted development of bone marrow or stem cell transplantation for cancer, and finally the series of events leading to the birth of the German Stammzellgesetz, or Stem Cell Act.

These stories illustrate how advances in stem cell and genomic research presented situations where ethical considerations are called for. They are examples of how modern advances in medicine have confronted patients, medical professionals, health-care providers, scientists, and society at large with issues that affect character formation, ethical education, and communication of values.

Heidelberg and New Orleans, 1985

Mr. S. D. was the CEO of the German branch of an international bank. He was a commanding, self-confident figure and had his life and the people around him always under control. In 1984, at the age of fifty-two, he was diagnosed with multiple myeloma (MM). After several failed treatment attempts, he came to our Heidelberg Medical Center in September of 1985. Bedridden at presentation and hardly able to move without excruciating pain, he was immediately hospitalized and received another treatment cycle of chemotherapy, which did not improve his situation.

As he heard that I was traveling to the Twenty-Seventh Annual Meeting of the American Society for Hematology (ASH) in New Orleans, Louisiana (December 7 to 10, 1985) to give a presentation, he came up with an extraordinary idea. The annual meeting of ASH is the premier event for hematologists worldwide. The most advanced and novel treatment results are presented by leaders in the field. The world's best hematologists will all come to New Orleans, he reasoned; why can't I gather the experts in MM and request their opinion on the treatment of my disease? He invited fifteen leaders for a group consultation on his specific case the day before the official opening of the conference, with promise of a compensation of one thousand U.S. dollars for each participant. Twelve of the selected fifteen accepted his invitation and turned up at the group consultation in a noble hotel in New Orleans.

He himself was flown in on a private jet equipped for transporting paralytic patients from our hospital to New Orleans. It was unusual that twelve international experts, together with three physicians from our department in Heidelberg, all gathered around him at a round table and exchanged ideas on the most appropriate management. Every expert offered his opinion on favorite experimental drug or strategy. Only one of the experts, from Baltimore, advised him: "There is no treatment that holds any meaningful promise. For the limited time that is left for you, you should not waste your resources to clutch at any straw but spend these valuable moments with your loved ones at home."

Mr. S. D. finally decided to go with the expert from MD Anderson Cancer Center, in Houston, Texas, who proposed a stem cell transplantation. This procedure was then a highly experimental treatment whose outcome was unknown.[1] He died within a few days after transferral, before any treatment could be initiated. He married his long-time girlfriend before dying.

This anecdote raises a number of questions that may be of interest for us:

1. Most experts have a propensity to come up with the "smartest" proposals in the name of medical advances, especially in a conference of professionals. They tend to clutch at every straw of experimental procedure that might promise a glimmer of success. This raises the ethical question of how far a patient with

---

[1] As of today, autologous blood stem cell transplantation has become a standard treatment for patients with multiple myeloma after they have achieved a very good remission, that is, after the cancer cells have been reduced drastically. In the case of multiple myeloma, the initial treatment consists of a combination of chemo- and immune therapy. High-dose chemotherapy may then induce a depletion of tumor cells and therefore a durable cure, but also cause irreversible toxicity to the blood stem cells in the bone marrow. By harvesting and storing the patient's own bone marrow (or hematopoietic stem cells) before high-dose chemotherapy, we could then induce a rapid recovery of blood formation by transplanting back the harvested bone marrow. Back in 1985, this strategy was highly experimental for multiple myeloma. The first series that showed some promise of success using high-dose melphalan with autologous bone marrow transplantation for multiple myeloma was published by B. Barlogie et al., "High-Dose Melphalan with Autologous Bone Marrow Transplantation for Multiple Myeloma," *Blood* 67 (1986): 1298–1301.

terminal disease should be encouraged to undergo another experimental treatment with unknown risks.

2. Very few medical experts—in this case only one—have the courage to provide realistic advice when confronted with a dying patient, especially one with adequate financial resources. This raises the question of character formation required for proper interaction with patients.

3. Some studies have shown that in every health care system in the "developed" world, a disproportionately large amount of health-care resources is spent on attempts to prolong life of patients who are terminally ill. This effectively reduces the resources for other patients or for other fields of health care—for example, health education. This raises the ethical question of proportionality and of what constitutes the appropriate allocation of resources.

4. In the everyday clinical environment, resources go beyond the availability of funds. They include human resources and the intensive engagement and commitment of health-care personnel all the time, twenty-four hours a day and seven days a week. How can we apply the principle of proportionality in the case of a dying patient? Can the extensive demand of resources be justified when the intensive care of one terminally ill patient effectively reduces the manpower and time needed for care of other patients?

San Diego, California, 1992

In August 1992, I was recruited by the University of California, San Diego (UCSD), to establish a stem cell transplantation program. Metastatic breast cancer was one of the innovative indications at the time.[2] Mrs. M. L., then forty-three

---

[2] As high-dose chemotherapy regimens succeeded in curing acute leukemia and Hodgkin's disease in the 1960 s, oncologists conjectured that solid tumors, such as breast cancer, might also respond to high-dose or megadose chemotherapy—for example, by quadrupling the dosage of drugs used conventionally. In the 1960 s, E. Donnall Thomas, at Fred Hutchinson Cancer Center in Seattle, Washington, and George Santos, at Johns Hopkins University, in Baltimore, Maryland, showed that bone marrow could be harvested from one patient and transplanted back—either into the same patient (autologous transplantation) or into another patient (allogeneic transplantation)—and restore the bone marrow function. For acute leukemia, this treatment principle of eliminating all leukemia cells, as well as all remaining normal cells in the bone marrow, and replacing it with healthy bone marrow from a compatible donor was phenomenally successful. In the case of allogeneic transplantation, the healthy immune system of the donor seems to play the dominant healing role. For his contribution, E. D. Thomas was honored with the Nobel Prize for Medicine and Physiology in 1990. In the case of autologous transplan-

years old, was one of the first patients in San Diego treated in a clinical trial.[3] After the procedure, she performed amazingly well and was free of any symptoms of disease. The treatment procedure and her personal interview filled two pages in the "Quest" section of the *San Diego Union Tribune* on March 10, 1993. The newspaper reporter communicated this complex procedure professionally and summarized his interview with the patient, focusing on the procedure from a patient's perspective. At the end of the interview, upon being told that the price tag amounted to $350,000 for the transplantation, he exclaimed: "Do you think that it is justified for society to spend so much resource on treatment of your disease, while this sum could have saved thousands of lives elsewhere in the world?" M. L. was very upset by this question.

The reporter's question was shocking to the patient. But it raised our awareness of a number of issues concerned.

1. Health and pursuit of happiness represent high values in our society. M. L. was young, and high-dose chemotherapy supported by blood stem cell transplant had become a treatment option for metastatic breast cancer in the late 1980 s and 1990 s.[4] She had excellent health insurance, and the insurance provider preapproved the treatment before we initiated the process. Many other patients in similar situations were denied this benefit by their insurance providers. The question here is, how can the balance in allocation of resources be maintained between the individual need to pursue health and the need of the community at large?

2. Stem cell transplant is an expensive procedure. In the United States, hospitals negotiate with insurance providers for a case rate for such high-cost treatment. Calculations are based not only on the recovery of expenses but also on the generation of revenue, as well as a reasonable profit margin for the treating

---

tation, the patient's own bone marrow was harvested, frozen, and transplanted back to induce a rapid reconstitution of bone marrow function.

[3] Clinical trials for cancer are research studies through which doctors find new ways to improve treatment results and the quality of life for patients with cancer. To render the results reproducible and to identify genuine benefits of a new drug or strategy, only patients who fulfill specific criteria for enrollment in a clinical trial are selected. With clinical trials, doctors are able to determine whether new treatments are safe and effective and work better than current standard treatments.

[4] In preliminary results from early-phase clinical trials, dose intensification is associated with superior outcomes in metastatic breast cancer. A few studies in the late 1980 s and early 1990 s showed that high-dose chemotherapy supported by autologous bone marrow transplantation could induce improvements in complete remission rates and long-term remission durations. Many clinical trials were subsequently activated in the United States and in Europe during this period.

institution. This raises the ethical question of how far financial gains should be based on people's suffering.

3. This case also raises the question of the costs of drugs and medication. What is a justified profit margin for patented drugs? One example is Lenalidomide, which is a modification of Thalidomide—the notorious drug used in the 1950 s and 1960 s for nausea and morning sickness for pregnant women. Thalidomide (trade name Contergan) caused dysmelia (malformation of limbs) in fetuses and was withdrawn from the market. In the 1990 s, with the discovery that Thalidomide and its derivative Lenalidomide are effective drugs for multiple myeloma, the cost of what used to be an inexpensive drug rose almost more than a hundredfold. A daily dose of Lenalidomide for treatment of multiple myeloma costs between $210 and $560, depending upon the country; patients should receive this drug daily for three weeks every month and continue treatment for months or sometimes years. What is a reasonable profit margin for the pharmaceutical industry?

Metastatic Breast Cancer—The Promise of Megadose Chemotherapy and Transplantation

In connection with the advanced breast cancer of Mrs. M. L., it is also appropriate to illustrate how convoluted the pursuit of scientific truth has turned out to be. The specific issue was whether high-dose, or megadose, chemotherapy and autologous transplantation are beneficial for metastatic breast cancer. The history of development of this innovative treatment principle revealed also how the premature promise of medical breakthrough affects ethical behavior of patients and doctors.

The worldwide enthusiasm for high-dose chemotherapy with autologous transplantation for patients with metastatic breast cancer lasted from the mid-1980 s to the 1990 s. The initial clinical trials, "Solid Tumor Autologous Marrow Program (STAMP)," pioneered by William (Bill) Peters and Emil Frei in 1982, at Dana Farber Cancer Institute, in Boston, Massachusetts, showed some promising trends by the end of 1984. The early phase clinical trials were intended to estimate the safety (Phase I study) and the potential efficacy (Phase II study) of a then novel treatment principle. The preliminary results were so encouraging that, once communicated at scientific conferences in the mid-1980 s, they aroused worldwide interest. Based on the initial data, Bill Peters and Emil Frei worked appropriately on a randomized (so-called Phase III) trial, in which patients would be assigned, at the flip of a coin, either to receiving megadose chemotherapy with autologous transplantation support, or to receiving conventional chemotherapy for metastatic breast cancer. Such Phase III trials are regarded as a litmus test to determine whether a novel treatment strategy is superior to conventional treatment.

In 1987, the initiation of this Phase III trial was finally approved and supported by the Cancer and Leukemia Group B (CALGB).[5] However, other oncologists from North America, the United Kingdom, France, and elsewhere already assumed that the STAMP regimen was so effective that they did not wait for the outcome of the Phase III trial. In this atmosphere, high-dose chemotherapy with bone marrow transplant became a big business for many oncology centers. Some insurance providers insisted, correctly, that this procedure was not yet of proven benefit and only "investigational," that is, not eligible for coverage by health insurance. Many patients in the United States who were denied the benefits of undergoing high-dose chemotherapy and transplantation filed lawsuits against their insurance providers, and in almost half of the cases the patients won. In late 1993, the Massachusetts state legislature even enacted a law that mandated coverage for transplantation for eligible patients within the state. Seven other states followed suit by the mid-1990 s.

Paradoxically, this development jeopardized immensely the scientific evaluation of the ongoing Phase III clinical trials. Everyone—that is, oncologists, advocacy groups, and insurance providers—supported the randomized Phase III clinical trials in principle, but most patients did not want to be enrolled in a randomized clinical trial, for fear that they might be assigned to the conventional chemotherapy arm. They opted for treatment using megadose and transplantation outside of the randomized trial.

One of the most prominent transplant promoters worldwide was Dr. W. B., in Johannesburg, South Africa. At a conference in Atlanta, in 1999, W. B. reported a phenomenally successful rate of nearly 60 percent of the patients in the transplant arm at the follow-up period of eight and a half years, versus 20 percent in the control. In contrast, interim reports from three other randomized trials showed equivocal results at the same oncology conference. With the consent of Dr. W. B., a team of American investigators traveled to Johannesburg to review the data and the patients' charts in 1999. The whole clinical trial of Dr. W. B. turned out to be a fraud, and this unique investigation was published in *Lancet*.[6] The misbehavior of an eminent oncologist fabricating positive results dealt a detrimental blow to the supporters of high-dose therapy for breast cancer and to the scientific community in general. In the subsequent months and years, contrary to initial expectations, the reports of randomized trials that compared

---

[5] CALGB is the centralized group that functions as a clearinghouse for clinical trials in the United States.

[6] The report of the American team investigating Dr. Bezwoda's study was published in Raymond B. Weiss et al., "High-Dose Chemotherapy for High-Risk Primary Breast Cancer: An On-Site Review of the Bezwoda Study," *Lancet* 355 (2000): 999–1003.

control groups with high-dose chemotherapy plus autologous transplantation have all shown negative outcomes—that is, high-dose chemotherapy has little or no benefit over conventional treatment regarding overall survival rates.[7]

This dramatic development within seventeen years of pursuit for better outcomes in a relatively common cancer disease has demonstrated the complexity of modern medicine and stem cell research, and the impact of premature communication of scientific advance on ethical behavior—for example, readiness to litigate. The scientific pathway to lasting improvements is littered with many pitfalls and is above all extremely time-consuming. A treatment principle such as stem cell transplantation that has worked excellently for leukemia and lymphoma may not work for patients with breast cancer. Carried away by encouraging results with transplantations for some cancer types in the 1980 s and 1990 s, many oncologists, and especially patients, were convinced that the novel strategy with high-dose chemotherapy and transplantation is also superior for breast cancer. Despite all the high hopes, expectations, and pressure from different levels of society, randomized trials did not show any long-term benefit. After seventeen years and fifteen Phase III clinical trials performed worldwide, the final evaluations showed unanimously a negative conclusion.[8] The most gratifying outcome from these years of frustration for all parties involved is the vindication that properly conducted research is paramount to establish truth and efficacy of novel treatments.

Heidelberg and Berlin, 2002–07

The next story revolves around stem cell research, and the series of events that led to the establishment of the first and second Stammzellgesetz—that is, laws and regulations that govern the use of human embryonic stem cell lines for scientific research in Germany.

Research in stem cells began in the early 1960 s. Ernest McCulloch, James Till, and Lou Siminovic, at the Ontario Cancer Institute, were the first scientists

---

[7] See W. P. Peters et al., "Prospective, Randomized Comparison of High-Dose Chemotherapy with Stem-Cell Support versus Intermediate-Dose Chemotherapy after Surgery and Adjuvant Chemotherapy in Women with High-Risk Primary Breast Cancer: A Report of CALGB 9082, SWOG 9114, and NCIC MA-13," *Journal of Clinical Oncology* 23 (2005): 2191–200; and D. A. Berry et al., "High-Dose Chemotherapy with Autologous Stem-Cell Support as Adjuvant Therapy in Breast Cancer: Overview of 15 Randomized Trials," *Journal of Clinical Oncology* 29 (2011): 3214–23.

[8] Berry et al., "High-Dose Chemotherapy with Autologous Stem-Cell Support as Adjuvant Therapy in Breast Cancer."

who defined the key properties of a stem cell.[9] They were the first to discover the blood-forming stem cells, (hematopoietic stem cells, HSC) in their pioneer work in mice. Since then, stem cells have been defined as cells that are able to self-renew and to differentiate into mature cell types. Such tissue-specific stem cells are referred to as multipotent—that is, they give rise to multiple cell types within a tissue or organ, and are essential for organ maintenance and repair in the living organism. Research using somatic or tissue-specific stem cells was not considered controversial.

As mentioned above, many patients with leukemia, lymphoma, and other diseases of the bone marrow owe their lives to advances in bone marrow transplantation, performed since the mid-1960 s. Our group in Heidelberg has shown that stem cells "mobilized" by specific drugs could be used instead of bone marrow, and that these mobilized stem cells were able to shorten the recovery time after transplantation by half. Because of this advantage, blood stem cells are the preferred source for transplantation nowadays.[10]

The establishment of human embryonic stem cell (hESC) lines at the end of 1998 has triggered worldwide interest and controversial debates around stem cell research.[11] Hopes soared high that pluripotent stem cells of human origin could represent sources of spare parts for all types of organs to replace diseased ones and might therefore play a major role in regenerative medicine. The bone of contention was that these cell lines originated from early human embryos.

In Germany as well as in many countries in the Western world, human embryos are protected by law (Embryonen-Schutz-Gesetz in Germany, passed on January 1, 1991).[12] Primarily the intention was to regulate what doctors and scientists are permitted to perform with the then novel technology in reproductive medicine. The aim was to protect human life and dignity and to prevent abuse of embryos by scientists and researchers. One major controversial issue is that, under this law, an embryo is defined as the fusion product of the nuclei of the egg cell with a sperm. Therefore, according to this law, human life begins already with fertilization.

Scientifically, fertilization of an egg cell by a sperm cell generates a zygote, the ultimate stem cell from which a living organism—for example, a human be-

---

[9] E. A. McCulloch and J. E. Till, "The Radiation Sensitivity of Normal Mouse Bone Marrow Cells, Determined by Quantitative Marrow Transplantation into Irradiated Mice," *Radiation Research* 13 (1960): 115-25.

[10] A. D. Ho, "Evolution of Peripheral Blood Stem Cell Transplantation," in *Stem Cell Mobilization: Methods and Protocols*, ed. Gerd Klein and Patrick Wuchter (New York: Humana Press, 2019), 1-10.

[11] J. A. Thomson et al., "Embryonic Stem Cell Lines Derived from Human Blastocysts," *Science* 282 (1998):1145-47.

[12] https://www.gesetze-im-internet.de/eschg/BJNR027460990.html.

ing—may derive. This stem cell has the potential to develop, after a myriad of divisions, into all organs and tissues of the body and is described as totipotent. In reality, a fertilized egg divides and develops into a blastocyst during the transport through the fallopian tube, which takes some two to four days. On days five to six, the cell number reaches thirty-two; the inner cell mass develops into the embryoblast, and the outer cells into the so-called trophoblast. On days seven to nine, and through the cells of the trophoblast that ultimately develops into the placenta, the blastocyst is embedded into the endometrium, a process called nidation. The inner cell mass consists of embryonic stem cells that are described as pluripotent. Only then can the blastocyst develop further into a fetus. Recent technologies show that approximately one-third to one-half of the eggs are able to reach the stage of nidation in humans.

Provided with the technologies to establish hESC lines in 1998, and with the potential to generate organs and tissues to replace diseased ones, hopes soared that embryonic stem cells might represent a source of cure for patients with various degenerative diseases that have not been treatable.

The opponents of hESC research claimed that embryos are sacrificed for the generation of such cell lines, and that this is forbidden by the Embryonen-Schutz-Gesetz. The reality is, however, that only half of the fertilized eggs—that is, embryos as defined by law—survive the journey from the fallopian tubes to the endometrium of the uterus. This controversy of when human life begins, and when an embryo acquires human dignity worthy to be protected under the Embryonen-Schutz-Gesetz, has led to numerous discussions at all levels of society.

Since establishment of hESC lines at the end of 1998, there have been heated debates in Germany and unprecedented public discussions on the ethics of human embryonic stem cell research, engaging politicians, religious leaders, lawyers, medical professionals, and society at large. On March 29, 2000, a status seminar initiated by the Federal Ministry of Education and Research brought together leaders from politics, law, ethics, and biological and medical sciences to deliberate on the status of stem cell and genome research and respective regulations. This kicked off many rounds of discussion initiated by diverse public and private organizations in Germany around the ethics of hESC research. Town hall meetings were hosted at the federal, state, community, and university levels.

Numerous public and private organizations—for example, the Adenauer Foundation, the Friedrich-Ebert Foundation, and the Kolping Foundation—delved into the discussion with impulse lectures and round-table sessions. I myself was involved in many round-table discussions and pleasantly surprised by how well informed most of the lawmakers involved in such discussions were. Finally, with a narrow margin, the first version of the Stammzell-Gesetz (StZGes) was passed in the Federal Parliament on July 1, 2002, permitting the import of human embryonic stem cell lines for scientific research of "high relevance."[13] A Central Ethics Commission (ZES) for human embryonic stem cell research was established to review the ethical and scientific merits of all applications as mandated by the StZGes.[14] The members of the ZES—two representatives from biology, three from medicine, two from ethics, and two from theology—have emphasized the significance of interactions between ethics and biomedical science in this process.[15]

The first version of this law was also unique, in that an expiry date of the legislation was set, providing opportunity for reassessment of the law after five years. A modification was indeed introduced on May 1, 2007, and finally passed on August 21, 2008. It was gratifying to see that many members of parliament who voted against the initial version of the law in 2002 changed their opinion, such that the second version of the law in 2008 was passed with a large majority.

In the developments that led to the passing and review of the StZG, the following points are relevant to our discussion:

1. Advances in medicine have generated the urgent need for interdisciplinary discussions on the scientific and appropriate use of new technologies. Medicine alone cannot and should not come up with the ethical norms for treatment, but it certainly presented a situation where they needed to be discussed and challenged. It was remarkable that politicians and lawmakers in Germany put a lot of effort into getting direct information from the scientists. For me, it was a unique learning experience to participate in interactions among politicians, scientists, church leaders, philosophers, and lawyers and to understand their viewpoints. This story shows how fruitful interdisciplinary discussions have led to a reasonable consensus and to a legislature that permits scientific advance under consideration of ethical concerns.

2. A central question within all these debates has been, when does life begin? Although a definite answer has yet to be found, I prefer the understanding that life begins when the fertilized egg comes to nidation and hence to direct interaction with the mother. In analogy, as advances in biomedicine progress, the question of when life ends also becomes debatable. Furthermore, what is the proportionality of allocating resources for costly experimental treatment attempts for a terminally ill patient with minimal hope of success?

In July 2022, twenty years have passed since the first constitutive meeting of the ZES was held at the Robert-Koch-Institute in Berlin on July 11, 2002. Dur-

---

[13] https://www.gesetze-im-internet.de/stzg/__4.html.
[14] https://www.rki.de/DE/Content/Kommissionen/ZES/zes_node.html.
[15] https://www.rki.de/DE/Content/Kommissionen/ZES/Mitglieder/mitglieder_node.html.

ing this period, ninety-six studies using hESC lines have been approved.[16] The frank and open discussion sessions in the business meetings of the ZES, with detailed deliberation on every single application, have been a learning experience for members and attendees. Although a number of restrictions are associated with this law—for example, only hESC lines that were generated before May 1, 2007, could be imported, and while use of hESC for research to gain scientific knowledge is permitted, paradoxically it is not allowed for translation into clinical pharmaco-toxicologic application—this piece of legislature has made possible top research using hESC in Germany. This was reflected in the increase in the number of relevant publications from German institutions in the past twenty years. The interactions, and occasionally heated discussions, within the ZES dealing with the pros and cons of each application for the use of hESC lines have bridged some of the differences in opinion and have been a mutually rewarding experience.

The principle behind the cure using allogeneic stem cell transplantation has been shown to be the replacement of the defective immune system of a cancer patient by a healthy one. In the meantime, this knowledge has led to the next level of recent development—that is, in the use of genetically manipulated immune cells, specifically T-lymphocytes derived from the patient, but genetically "educated" in the laboratory to target tumor cells. After cultivation and expansion in the laboratory, these lymphocytes are given back to the patient to eradicate the corresponding tumor cells. The use of such genetically manipulated lymphocytes, called Chimeric Antigen Receptor T cells (CAR-T-cells), against specific tumor antigens has proven to be very effective for some cancer types.

As with all modern advances in biomedical research, these novel treatment strategies are labor- and cost-intensive. It is necessary to discuss the complex issues of allocation of resources in relation to expensive treatment for patients with little hope of cure. How do we maintain the balance between the allocation of resources for the common good and for the individual with his indisputable right to pursue life and happiness? As in the case of hESC research, these are issues that not only concern medical professionals and scientists but also pose challenges to ethical decision-making for society.

---

[16] Tätigkeitsbericht der Zentral Ethik-Kommission für Stammzellforschung (ZES). 19. Bericht nach Inkrafttreten des Stammzellgesetztes (StZG), https://www.rki.de/DE/Content/Kommissionen/ZES/Taetigkeitsberichte/19-taetigkeitsbericht.pdf?__blob=publicationFile.

The Acceptance of Genetic Technologies by Individuals, Societies, and Health-Care Systems

Ruth M. Farrell

Introduction

Advances in genomic science and technology have significantly impacted the delivery of reproductive health care. The newest tests can be used in prenatal care to help pregnant patients and families make informed decisions about their reproductive health and family-building efforts. At the same time, these technologies generate a series of unprecedented challenges for patients, families, and society. These challenges are due, in part, to the volume and complexity of information such technologies can produce, and in part to issues embedded in the nature and degree of uncertainty that comes with acquiring and determining the significance of fetal genomic information before birth. These challenges are also closely tied to medical, social, and legal constructs and how individuals can interface with them. To complicate matters, the pathway by which these technologies traverse from the bench to the bedside presents challenges of its own, a journey entrenched in the dynamics resulting from factors external to the interests of individuals and families.

This chapter examines the multifaceted aspects that affect the translation of genomics in the reproductive context, focusing on prenatal genetic screens and diagnostic tests (referred to in this chapter as prenatal genetic tests). These tests are a central component of the delivery of high-quality, evidence-based prenatal care.[1] They contribute to favorable obstetric outcomes, given that congenital ab-

---

[1] World Health Organization, "Birth Defects: Key Facts," Feb. 28, 2022, https://www.who.int/news-room/fact-sheets/detail/birth-defects; Ocilia Maria Costa Carvalho et al., "Delays in Obstetric Care Increase the Risk of Neonatal Near-Miss Morbidity Events and Death: A Case-Control Study," *BMC Pregnancy Childbirth* 20 (2020): 437, https://doi.org/10.1186/s12884-020-03128-y; and M. Michie, "Is Preparation a Good Reason for Prenatal Genetic Testing? Ethical and Critical Questions," *Birth Defects Research* 112, no. 4 (2020): 332–38, https://doi.org/10.1002/bdr2.1651.

normalities are a leading cause of infant mortality in the United States.[2] Annually, more than four thousand infants in the United States die within their first year of life, due to congenital abnormalities, and those who survive beyond this time are more likely to have long-term health conditions that impact their quality of life and the lives of their families.[3] This is particularly true for those who experience delays in diagnosing and managing these disorders. The information gained from prenatal genetic tests may inform significant decisions during the pregnancy: the possibility of additional antenatal evaluations or maternal-fetal procedures to manage complications; interventions during labor and delivery (for example, induction of labor, cesarean section); arrangements for specialty pediatric care after birth; or coordinating household, health care, and financial preparations for a child with medical needs. If a serious condition is diagnosed, this information may lead to the decision to end the pregnancy, which is associated with increasing uncertainties about access to abortion services. Given the ramifications of these decisions for the patient and family, it is a priority to ensure that the needs, goals, and values of pregnant women drive decisions about whether to use these tests, which testing approach to use (for example, screening tests vs. diagnostic tests), and when in the pregnancy to utilize them.

With these considerations in mind, decisions about use of prenatal genetic testing should focus on the values, needs, and goals of pregnant women and their families. However, in reality, those decisions are heavily influenced by social systems that affect not just the existence of technology to identify a fetal variant but also the expectations and beliefs about obtaining that information during pregnancy and then acting on it. Thus, there is a complex interplay of

---

[2] K. Lee et al., "Infant Mortality from Congenital Malformations in the United States, 1970-1997," *Obstetrics & Gynecology* 98, no. 4 (2001): 620-27, https://doi.org/10.1016/S0029-7844(01)01507-1.

[3] American Academy of Pediatrics, American College of Obstetricians and Gynecologists, *Guidelines for Perinatal Care* (Washington, DC: American Academy of Pediatrics and American College of Obstetricians and Gynecologists, 2012); K. Lee et al., "Infant Mortality from Congenital Malformations in the United States"; A. Gadson, E. Akpovi, and P. K. Mehta, "Exploring the Social Determinants of Racial/Ethnic Disparities in Prenatal Care Utilization and Maternal Outcome," *Seminars in Perinatology* 41, no. 5 (2017): 308-17; Centers for Disease Control, "Data & Statistics on Birth Defects," 2020, https://www.cdc.gov/ncbddd/birthdefects/data.html; J. Xu et al., "Deaths: Final Data for 2013," *National Vital Statistics Reports* 64, no. 2 (2016):1-119; L. M. Almli et al., "Infant Mortality Attributable to Birth Defects—United States, 2003-2017," *Morbidity and Mortality Weekly Report* 69, no. 2 (2020):25-29, https://doi.org/10.15585/mmwr.mm6902a1; and S. Glinianaia et al., "Long-Term Survival of Children Born with Congenital Anomalies: A Systematic Review and Meta-Analysis of Population-Based Studies," *PLOS Medicine* 7, no. 9 (2020), https://doi.org/10.1371/journal.pmed.1003356.

social systems that impact both actionability and agency during pregnancy, with significant implications for the pregnant person, their family, community, society, and future generations. In this chapter, I consider how social systems influence actionability and agency, as well as the challenges that patients must navigate to ensure that their choices about prenatal genetic technologies reflect who they are as individuals and as members of families and communities.

Prenatal Genetic Technologies and Actionability

Actionability is a critical topic to address when considering the development and use of prenatal genetic tests. In this section, I consider actionability in the sense of actions made available for a patient to use or decline during pregnancy. To fully understand actionability in this context, I first develop a foundational basis for understanding these technologies in order to explore their significance for patients, families, and communities.

Prenatal genetic screens constitute one group of options available to pregnant women. Screens provide information about the risk of a fetal genetic condition. While they cannot produce a definitive answer about the presence or absence of a condition, their benefit lies in their ability to help inform decisions about additional testing that might be needed during the pregnancy. Furthermore, screening tests are performed by sampling maternal blood or through an ultrasound. For this reason, they do not pose significant risks to the fetus. Before recent advances in molecular genetics, prenatal maternal serum screens (for example, the triple screen or quadruple screen) analyzed a series of biomarkers in the maternal serum to obtain risk information about a limited number of conditions. These conditions included the common autosomal aneuploidies—that is, Trisomy 21 (Down syndrome), Trisomy 18 (Edwards syndrome), and Trisomy 13 (Patau syndrome)—as well as neural tube defects.

While maternal serum screens provide risk information about the fetus, they are associated with significant rates of false positive and false negative results. As a result, further diagnostic testing is needed to confirm the presence of any condition identified in the screen. Subsequent advances in biotechnology led to the development of cell-free DNA screening (cfDNA), a molecular-based screen that is better able to identify Trisomy 21, Trisomy 18, and Trisomy 13 and has a lower risk of false positive results. In addition, cfDNA can provide information about a series of other chromosomal variants (for example, sex chromosome aneuploidies) and genomic variants (for example, microdeletions, duplications), vastly increasing the number and type of variants that can be identified before birth.[4] There is also growing interest in using cfDNA to provide information about single-gene disorders, marking a significant evolution in this technology.

Despite these improvements, cfDNA is a screening test, not a diagnostic test. Thus, there is still an essential role for prenatal diagnostic tests, as they can provide definitive information about the presence or absence of a genetic variant. Currently, two diagnostic tests are available: chorionic villus sampling, which is performed in the first trimester of pregnancy, and amniocentesis, which is performed in the second trimester. Both of these are invasive procedures that involve inserting a needle into the uterus and retrieving cells from the placenta or the amniotic fluid, which is then analyzed to identify a variant. While conventional analysis techniques (for example, fluorescent in situ hybridization, or FISH) are used to identify numerical or structural chromosomal abnormalities, it is now possible to identify hundreds of other fetal genomic variants, including copy-number variants, through cytogenetic microarray analysis and other molecular-based techniques that are currently being developed.[5] However, while there is now a vast increase in the amount of overall data that can be obtained through analysis, the ability to interpret this data lags far behind. In addition, invasive diagnostic procedures carry the risk of miscarriage and other obstetric complications. While such risks are low, they shape how patients and providers view the advantages and disadvantages of these procedures.

Considering the remarkable scientific advances that have led to prenatal genetic tests, it is necessary also to consider broader questions of actionability beyond the specific tests available, as well as the goals and intentions of prenatal genetic testing technology. This leads to a central set of questions related to actionability: What social systems and imagined worlds have led to developing the ability to learn about the genetic composition of a fetus before birth? How have these systems served as a driver to developing and implementing the technologies used to obtain this information? Considering these questions includes asking why it has been made possible to gain genetic information about the fetus in the first place, and why certain conditions have been chosen as ones that should be identified in that process.

---

[4] R. M. Farrell, B. Nutter, and P. K. Agatisa, "Patient-Centered Prenatal Counseling: Aligning Obstetric Healthcare Professionals with the Needs of Pregnant Women," *Women & Health* 55 (2015): 280–96.

[5] National Society of Genetic Counselors, "Prenatal Cell-Free DNA Screening," 2021, https://www.nsgc.org/Policy-Research-and-Publications/Position-Statements/Position-Statements/Post/prenatal-cell-free-dna-screening-1; and B. Zimmermann et al., "Noninvasive Prenatal Aneuploidy Testing of Chromosomes 13, 18, 21, X, and Y, Using Targeted Sequencing of Polymorphic Loci," *Prenatal Diagnosis* 32 (2012): 1233–41, doi: 10.1002/pd.3993.

It is well-recognized that scientific development does not occur in a vacuum. Instead, science and scientific discovery are a function of societal values and how those values manifest in the direction and pace of scientific discovery. Those societal values, in turn, establish the parameters for what may be considered "good" versus "bad," "right" versus "wrong," or "acceptable" versus "unacceptable" uses of the technology. Additionally, a myriad of social systems contributes to individual and collective perceptions of other fundamental concepts, such as the notions of health, disease, and disability, in addition to diversity and inclusion. How these concepts are established goes beyond the influence of values with respect to gaining genetic information about the fetus. The advances that have led to new prenatal genetic tests have been affected by values around scientific progress and intellectual property. Over the past decade, commercial laboratories have been predominant in developing, marketing, and implementing new screens and diagnostic tests. This trend, positioned to continue in the coming years, calls for questioning who will gain if these tests are broadly implemented across the pregnant patient population.

Behind this line of inquiry are larger questions about the goals of this technology, and the outcomes that signal that those goals have been achieved. These questions include questions about what kind of world these technologies are intended to create, based on what kinds of societal beliefs about the capability of human existence, quality of life, diversity, and both individual and collective agency. These questions in turn lead to a discussion about agency, the choices of individuals to use or decline tests, and whether and how the tests may be part of larger technological development goals.

Prenatal Genetic Technologies and Agency

Knowing that the option of prenatal genetic testing exists, what agency does an individual have to use those technologies to actualize a pathway aimed at achieving their goals, needs, and values with respect to self, pregnancy, parenthood, and family? Such agency should manifest as the informed and voluntary decision to use such technologies in a way that aligns with the patient's values about what steps to take if a fetal genetic condition is diagnosed. Agency thus includes the option either to decline or to pursue testing if the information gained or experiences of the process are discordant with the patient's needs and goals as a pregnant individual and parent. These choices resonate not just around the individual's considerations about the significance of a genetic condition, what it may mean for a child, and what steps may be elected to avoid or allow that outcome; such choices also concern the tolerance of uncertainty. This includes beliefs about the value assigned to knowing or not knowing about a fetal genetic variant before birth, the degree of uncertainty that patients are willing to accept in that process, and the gains that they perceive will come from remaining in a state of uncertainty. For some, uncertainty takes the form of declining prenatal genetic testing. For others who choose prenatal genetic testing, the quest for certainty may nevertheless lead to an uncertain path, as such tests do not necessarily eliminate questions and may instead raise many others. Thus, while definitive information is available about what options exist, the social forces associated with whether, when, and how to use such options are entrenched in factors that may either support agency or erode it.

Agency as a Function of Scientific and Clinical Uncertainty

There are many uncertainties associated with the science of genetics and genomics,[6] as the detection of a genetic variant cannot predict outcomes for an individual. The rate at which new tests have emerged has outpaced our scientific understanding of what the results may mean. This is particularly true in prenatal genetic testing, where detailed phenotypic and clinical information is unavailable until after birth. Despite advances in genomic science, there remains uncertainty about how mild or significant a variant may be and how that variant may impact the quality of life for a child. Instead, forecasting a picture of future health and well-being is a calculus of probability based on what may be determined from other antenatal procedures, such as sonography. This information may be most accurate for the most common conditions, leaving unanswered questions about the outcomes for children and adults with rare conditions and genomic variants of uncertain significance. While scientific and medical information can be applied in prenatal care, accurate information about how a genetic condition may manifest is unavailable until after birth. In addition, with the growth of molecular methods to conduct genomic analysis, it is possible to identify variation that is not fully understood. For instance, there is a series of genetic variants called variants of uncertain significance (VUS) for which we need to learn what they may mean, either by themselves or when those genes interact with others or with environmental exposures.

Increasing uncertainty is not due merely to advances in prenatal genetics. It is also due to the shifting options available to pregnant patients if a fetal genetic condition is diagnosed. There are also increasing uncertainties about what steps a pregnant patient may take if a condition is diagnosed. This factor is directly related to short-term and long-term outcomes for the pregnant person after pregnancy. These questions consider the efficacy and safety of postdiagnosis inter-

---

[6] Genetics is the study of heredity and variations in inherited characteristics. Genomics is the study of the structure, function, variation, evolution, and mapping of genomes.

ventions and access to the highest-quality health care to receive those interventions. Until recently, the options for patients if a fetal genetic condition was confirmed were primarily limited to either preparation and anticipatory guidance for the birth of a child with a potentially serious medical condition (for example, coordinating obstetric and neonatal management plans, arranging household and financial resources) or ending the pregnancy, with only limited interventions available to improve outcomes. These options were made more complex by the existence of barriers inhibiting patients' ability to access information and resources. This situation is rapidly becoming even more complex, given recent changes in maternal-fetal medicine, neonatology, and reproductive medicine.

On one hand, there is the growth and development of new postdiagnosis interventions: advances in maternal-fetal medicine, neonatology, and pediatrics are making significant inroads toward improving outcomes for infants with congenital conditions.[7] In addition, there is a growing interest in trials that can provide data on interventions to mitigate the downstream impact of a genetic condition on development.[8] On the other hand, patients have diminishing options if they decide to end the pregnancy. In the United States, increasing restrictions on abortions raise concerns about a patient's ability to access abortion services if a severe fetal genetic condition is identified. There is a powerful immediacy required for each of these decisions—whether to terminate the pregnancy or to pursue interventions to improve outcomes for the newborn.

Given the pace and trajectory of medical science, it is also essential to consider options that may be available in the near future. These may include medical breakthroughs that could change the life course of an individual with a genetic condition. One significant uncertainty is whether treatment could be developed that would mitigate the effect of certain genetic conditions. In our current health paradigms, this could be a medical or surgical treatment that could improve quality of life. It is also essential to consider a major shift in reproductive genetics and genomics. Traditionally, genomic science focused on genetic screening and diagnostic testing. However, the focus is increasingly on interventions in the human genome, epigenome, or microbiome. For instance, researchers are increasingly focusing on ways to modify genetic material, aiming to "correct a problem" or, in some cases, to "enhance" the function or health of a child.[9] The recent births of children whose genomes were modified at the embryonic

---

[7] Xu et al., "Deaths: Final data for 2013"; Almli et al., "Infant Mortality Attributable to Birth Defects"; and Glinianaia et al., "Long-Term Survival of Children Born with Congenital Anomalies."
[8] World Health Organization, "Birth Defects: Key Facts."
[9] American Academy of Pediatrics, American College of Obstetricians and Gynecologists, "Guidelines for Perinatal Care."

stage highlight both rapid advancement in genome modification and serious ethical and social implications stemming from this new frontier in genomics.[10]

A medical framework does not by itself construct the concept of outcomes for an individual with a genetic condition. While science can provide some empirical data about the degree of function or dysfunction of different anatomical and physiological functions in a child and adult, how that individual will fare in childhood and throughout their life is a function of societal values. In part, that is a function of the physical and social infrastructure that enables differently abled individuals to interact within communities. These values, in turn, establish systems that are in place to support persons with a genetic condition and the families who care for them. Thus, the severity of a condition may be significantly influenced by the presence or absence of resources and structures that support functioning at home and in communities. It is also a function of how values may change over time, with the recognition and acceptance of diversity manifested in how social structures may increase or restrict the resources and levels of inclusivity for individuals with a genetic condition and individuals in communities.

Agency as a Function of Access

Agency is also a function of a patient's ability to learn about their prenatal genetic testing options and make an informed decision about their use. Given the complexity and ramifications of decisions about prenatal genetic tests for patients and families, systems must be in place to ensure that patients have the information they need to make informed decisions that reflect their decision-making preferences, tolerance of uncertainty, values, and beliefs. As it currently stands, U.S. health policy recommends that all patients should be offered prenatal genetic testing regardless of their age, race, or reproductive history. In the context of this option, patients consider whether to use the technology or decline it. There are significant implications for the pregnant patient, the fetus, and the patient's family with either of these choices. Thus, it is critical that pregnant patients be able to manifest their agency through informed decision-making.

The ability to make a voluntary and informed decision is a function of the patient's familiarity with concepts associated with genetics, including the notions of risk and probability. For patients and their families, decision-making may begin with questions about how the different prenatal genetic tests may work, what conditions they may provide information about, and how accurate

---

[10] Almli et al., "Infant Mortality Attributable to Birth Defects"; Glinianaia et al., Long-Term Survival of Children Born with Congenital Anomalies"; World Health Organization, "Congenital Anomalies"; Carvalho et al., "Delays in Obstetric Care Increase the Risk of Neonatal Near-Miss Morbidity."

the results will be, given the chance of false positive and false negative results. However, studies demonstrate that expectant parents face several challenges in obtaining accurate, unbiased information and decisional support that reflects their needs when navigating their prenatal genetic testing options.[11] For example, while many patients may be familiar with common autosomal aneuploidies, such as Trisomy 21, they have little knowledge of sex chromosome aneuploidies and significantly less knowledge of microdeletion syndromes and other genomic variants.[12] Persistent issues related to low health literacy and knowledge of genetics, risk, and probability lie at the foundation of the problem.[13]

Uncertainty is also a function of the information presented to patients about their options. Studies show that obstetric providers face numerous barriers to providing personalized, effective, and patient-centered counseling about some of the newest prenatal genetic tests and have limited resources to meet the needs of a diverse population of patients with varying degrees of health literacy and knowledge of different genetic conditions, as well as different beliefs about parenthood, disability, and pregnancy termination. This challenge is due, in part, to clinicians themselves having varied knowledge of and experience with prenatal genetic tests, and particularly with the performance and interpretation of complex panel tests. It is also due to the ability of a health-care provider to convey information about the testing options in a way that patients can comprehend. To do so, information delivery (of the knowns and unknowns of a genetic condition) must be accurate, unbiased, and timely, so that patients may make informed choices about their testing options in early pregnancy, during the window for possible antenatal intervention. However, this process may be plagued by conscious and unconscious bias and assumptions by a clinician about what information a patient may desire and the choices they may make in light of that information. The process is also a function of information available through media, marketing, and social messages about the acceptability or unacceptability of using these tests to identify a fetal genetic variant. Currently, many commercial laboratories that develop new prenatal genetic tests also take the lead in marketing and media messages about the genetic conditions that can be identified and the value of using technology to identify those conditions.

---

[11] M. Kuppermann et al., "Effect of Enhanced Information, Values Clarification, and Removal of Financial Barriers on Use of Prenatal Genetic Testing: A Randomized Clinical Trial," *JAMA* 312, no. 12 (Sep. 24, 2014):1210–17, doi: 10.1001/jama.2014.11479.

[12] Zimmermann et al., "Noninvasive Prenatal Aneuploidy Testing."

[13] M. E. Norton et al., "Non-Invasive Chromosomal Evaluation (NICE) Study: Results of a Multicenter Prospective Cohort Study for Detection of Fetal Trisomy 21 and Trisomy 18," *American Journal of Obstetrics and Gynecology* 207, no. 2 (2012): 137.e1–8. Doi: 10.1016/j.ajog.2012.05.021.

Agency is not only a function of the ability to access health care and medical technology. It is also a function of whether and when during pregnancy a patient will access health care and a health-care provider who can offer this information. Structural, systemic, and environmental factors are known to affect the ability to access prenatal care early in pregnancy and are associated with adverse obstetric outcomes. In addition, agency is a function of insurers, who dictate the out-of-pocket expenses for insurance coverage of tests and prenatal and postnatal options for acting on information, including access to specialty and fertility care centers where innovative care can be received.

Agency and Personal Uncertainty

Beyond the scientific and clinical aspects of identifying a fetal variant, there is also the personal uncertainty of what action to take in light of the consequences of a decision to use or decline prenatal genetic testing. Such existential uncertainty pertains to how an individual may view themselves in the world and how the world in which they exist gives context to the meaning and significance of using or declining tests that provide fetal genetic information during pregnancy. These are profound yet frequently unexplored considerations. For some, the offer of prenatal genetic testing is the first time they may confront fundamental questions about agency and actionability as they consider beliefs about the quality of life, the value of knowledge, and tolerance of uncertainty during pregnancy. For others, these questions may have been explored earlier in life (for example, separate from or in conjunction with an earlier pregnancy or shared life experiences of family and friends) but bring on new levels of uncertainty in the context of the current pregnancy with the specific medical and life circumstances surrounding it.

There is also the uncertainty about what an individual parent or family may do to optimize the quality of life for a child with a genetic condition. In the context of reproductive medicine, it is essential to consider the family and how they may perceive the severity of a child's condition with respect to what resources they can commit to the care of a child with a genetic condition. Uncertainty may also stem from the dynamic nature of a family and how the family may change over time. For instance, the addition of more children may bring the possibility that others will also require resources for a medical condition. The possible loss of a parent or parents raises the question of who will care for a child or adult with a genetic condition, and whether that individual can be cared for at home or must be transferred to a skilled facility.

There is also the sense of internal change in perspective and adapting to life as it unfolds. This is an experience felt by many patients who face a challenge that may seem insurmountable, but who then discover that, when taken in incremental steps, it can be managed. Considerations may also extend the scope of the implications stemming from the decision to accept or decline prenatal genetic testing. The decision to act or not act may affect the individual and further decisions about the pregnancy. At the same time, the decision can have implications for the family with respect to its composition, dynamic, function, health, and well-being as well as that of the larger society. There may also be uncertainty about the ramifications of the decision over time, including the experiences during the pregnancy or later in the woman's life. It may also affect future generations, in which the presence or absence of a genetic variant may impact human existence. Each of these considerations is particularly relevant in prenatal genetic testing, where numerous variables must be considered before birth, and futures with or without a child with a genetic condition must be imagined using uncertain data.

Actionability, Agency, and Uncertainty

Advances in genetics and genomics have made a significant impact on prenatal care delivery. Yet in doing so, they prompt a series of questions and uncertainties about their existence and the implications of the decision to use or decline them during pregnancy. Given those uncertainties, it is vital to consider the interplay among actionability, uncertainty, and agency. While technologies for acquiring detailed genetic information about a fetus exist, there is no clear answer to the question of whether to use them to their fullest potential or to defer insight into outcomes until after birth. Those uncertainties are, in part, a construct of the boundaries and conflicts between social systems and the beliefs, values, and goals of individuals who must make that decision. Ultimately, the availability of prenatal genetic tests raises fundamental questions about how the choice presented by their existence may empower or disempower a patient to manifest their agency.

Ethical Discourse on Epigenetics and Genome Editing: The Risk of (Epi-)Genetic Determinism and Scientifically Controversial Basic Assumptions[1]

Karla Alex and Eva C. Winkler

1. Introduction

This chapter provides insight into the diverse ethical debates on genetics and epigenetics.

Much controversy surrounds debates about intervening into the germline genome of human embryos, with catchwords such as *genome editing, designer baby,* and *CRISPR/Cas*.[2] The idea that it is possible to design a child according to one's personal preferences is, however, a quite distorted view of what is actually possible with new gene technologies and gene therapies. These are much more limited than the *editing* and *design* metaphors suggest. Such metaphors are therefore highly problematic phrases in the context of new gene technologies, for two reasons. On one hand, to design a *child of choice* by modifying the genome would require modifying any gene of choice, which is more than can be

---

[1] This chapter originated from the philosophical subproject of the project "COMParative ASSessment of Genome- and Epigenome-Editing in Medicine: Ethical, Legal and Social Implications" (COMPASS-ELSI and COMPASS-ELSI 2.0), funded by the German Research Foundation (DFG – 409799774). The article was first published in German as K. Alex and E. C. Winkler, "Ethischer Diskurs zu Epigenetik und Genom-Editierung. Die Gefahr eines (epi-)genetischen Determinismus und naturwissenschaftlich strittiger Grundannahmen;" in *Fünfter Gentechnologiebericht. Sachstand und Perspektiven für Forschung und Anwendung* [Fifth Gene Technology Report], ed. B. Fehse et al. (Baden-Baden: Nomos, 2021), 299–323, https://doi.org/10.5771/9783748927242; the present is a slightly modified version of the German version; translation Karla Alex. We thank Gary S. Hauk for assistance with language proofreading.

[2] CRISPR: "Clustered Regularly Interspaced Short Palindromic Repeats"; Cas: "CRISPR associated enzymes." CRISPR/Cas is used in gene therapy to bind specifically to DNA and, in some cases, to modify it. This is a genetic engineering process that has its origins in forms of bacterial immune defense.

done with current gene technologies, such as CRISPR/Cas. On the other hand, a modification of genes would need to be enough to create any characteristic of choice in the future child. The latter presupposes the assumption of *genetic determinism*.[3] Moreover, the CRISPR/Cas technology can not only be used in a potentially therapeutic manner at the germline level. In addition, there is the (more likely) scenario of a future clinical therapeutic use of these new gene technologies for modifying the DNA sequence of other cells of the body (somatic genome editing). There is also the option of modifying the epigenome, that is, the spatial configuration of DNA (epigenome editing) (see table 1).

Like genetics and genome editing, epigenetics has been at the center of recent popular scientific[4] and ethical discourse[5] as well as scientific debates. The concept of epigenetics has given rise to very different notions of inheritability and responsibility for health,[6] which, however, are often based on scientifically controversial basic assumptions. That there continues to be *covert genetic determinism* in the form of *epigenetic determinism* (see table 2) in debates about epigenetics has been pointed out in ethical analyses of epigenetics.[7] Neither genetic

---

[3] The different terms (here also -*isms*) are explained in the following text; for an overview see also table 2.

[4] The term "popular scientific discourse" covers texts that present scientific topics in a form understandable by the general public—for example, media science texts or self-help books (in German, "Ratgeberliteratur") on health topics.

[5] Of course, ethics is also to be counted among the disciplines of humanities (and in German simply among the broader term "Wissenschaft," often translated as "science," albeit comprising sciences and humanities). In the present study, therefore, the use of the term "science" refers to natural science, unless otherwise stated.

[6] On epigenetics, see the publication *Epigenetik. Implikationen für die Lebens- und Geisteswissenschaften*, by the Berlin-Brandenburg Academy of Sciences and Humanities, edited by Jörn Walter and Anja Hümpel (Baden-Baden: Nomos, 2017). That work provides an intensive analysis of the concept of heredity in the context of epigenetics, which is much more extensive and differentiated than can be done in the present chapter. For a more detailed discussion of this important topic, we therefore refer to Walter and Hümpel, *Epigenetik*. For the scientific basis of epigenetics, see also J. Walter and N. Gasparoni, "Themenbereich Epigenetik. Von Zellidentitäten bis hin zu Krankheiten und Therapien," in *Fünfter Gentechnologiebericht. Sachstand und Perspektiven für Forschung und Anwendung*, ed. B. Fehse et al. (Baden-Baden: Nomos, 2021), 93–113; and A. Jawaid and I. Mansuy, "Generationsübergreifende Auswirkungen von Traumata. Implikationen für Individuen und Gesellschaft," in Fehse et al., *Fünfter Gentechnologiebericht*, 277–98.

[7] S. Schuol, "Widerlegt die Epigenetik den Gendeterminismus? Es kommt darauf an …," in *Epigenetik. Ethische, rechtliche und soziale Aspekte*, ed. R. Heil et al. (Wiesbaden: Springer, 2016), 45–58; S. Schuol, *Das regulierte Gen. Implikationen der Epigenetik für Biophilosophie und Bioethik* (Freiburg/Munich: Karl Alber, 2017); and M. R. Waggoner and

Tab. 1. Genome Editing and Epigenome Editing.

	Genome editing	Epigenome editing
Method	Changing the DNA sequence (base sequence): – of germline cells, e.g., in embryos (germline intervention), – or of somatic cells (somatic genome editing).	Changing the structure of DNA for the purpose of influencing the transcription of DNA in the cell ("reading") and gene expression (conversion of DNA into proteins): – usually of somatic cells (somatic epigenome editing).
Application / Use cases	– Treatment of genetic diseases, – e.g., hemoglobinopathies – (beta thalassemia, sickle cell disease …). – What are hemoglobinopathies? – Disturbance of the formation or function of the red blood pigment hemoglobin with sometimes severe symptoms.	– Treatment of epigenetic diseases, – e.g., imprinting disorders – (Prader-Willi syndrome, Angelman syndrome, …). – What are imprinting disorders? – Syndromes caused by incorrect "reading" of genes with a combination of neurological symptoms, growth and metabolic impairments.

Scientific background:
- Genome and epigenome editing are gene technological methods.
- As in genome editing, the "CRISPR/Cas complex" is frequently used in epigenome editing, other available "tools" are Zinc Finger Nucleases (ZFN) and "Transcription Activator-Like Effector Nucleases" (TALENs).
- However, the Cas enzyme, which is generally used in genome editing to induce DNA breakage, is modified in such a way that it is provided in the form of "catalytically deactivated-Cas" (dCas).
- The use of "CRISPR/dCas" in epigenome editing thus enables binding to DNA without causing DNA breakage.
- While genome editing changes the DNA sequence, epigenome editing aims to modify the epigenetic configuration of chromatin, e.g., DNA methylation change and histone acetylation change.

determinism nor epigenetic determinism has been confirmed scientifically. It is therefore important to recognize the concepts that are discussed (and sometimes harshly criticized) in debates about genome editing and epigenetics—for exam-

---

T. Uller, "Epigenetic Determinism in Science and Society," *New Genetics and Society* 34, no. 2 (2015): 177–95, DOI: 10.1080/14636778.2015.1033052.

ple, concepts about the causal role of DNA for our own life course. This importance is based on the fact that if we understand such controversial concepts, we will be able to remain critical when evaluating scientific knowledge and ethical arguments about genome editing and epigenetics. This chapter, therefore, explains some of these concepts. For an ethical analysis of epigenetics as well as of genome editing, it is necessary to understand and critically reflect upon the underlying concepts of genetic determinism and other, related *-isms*. The following section offers a detailed introduction to these -isms (section 2; see also table 2).

Section 3 provides an ethical analysis of genome editing and epigenetics based on the explanations in section 2. Section 3 focuses on inheritability and responsibility, justice, safety, the problem of consent, and the effects of genome editing and epigenetics on embryos and future generations.

This section does not discuss in detail further points that can be found in ethical debates about epigenetics as well as in ethical debates about genome editing. These points include (among others):
- fear that the findings of epigenetics and that the methods of genome editing are misused–this also with respect to eugenics and *enhancement*;[8]
- naturalness–an issue we mention in passing a few times in the following analysis;
- a possible connection between the genome/epigenome and the concept of human dignity, and the derived danger of instrumentalization and infringement of autonomy when intervening in the genome or epigenome.

Since current discourse about ethical issues associated with genome editing focuses mainly on germline interventions–which are, for instance, interventions into a human embryo's genome–we mainly focus on germline interventions when comparing the debates on genome editing and on epigenetics in section 3.

2. -isms

An important concern of this chapter is to draw attention to the need for critical reflection on explicit, but far more often implicit, -isms within the discourse on epigenetics as well as genetics and genome editing. The following concepts or -isms, which are highlighted to varying degrees in scientific, popular scientific, societal, and ethical discourse, will be discussed–namely, genetic essentialism and strong genetic determinism (2.1), covert genetic determinism and epigenet-

---

[8] See Dieter Birnbacher, "Gentechnisches Enhancement," in *Vierter Gentechnologiebericht. Bilanzierung einer Hochtechnologie* [Fourth Gene Technology Report], ed. F. Hucho et al. (Baden-Baden: Nomos, 2018), 237–50; see also below, section 3.1.

Tab. 2. Analyzed Concepts.

	Definition	Section	Related areas of discourse			
			Scien.	P.-Scien.	Soc.	Eth.
Genetic essentialism	Idea that a person is determined solely, or at least to a predominant part, by their genes.	2.1			X	
Strong genetic determinism	Idea that a gene almost always determines a certain characteristic (a particular physical, behavioral, or character trait).	2.1			X	
Covert genetic determinism	Adoption of genetic determinism extended by the findings of epigenetics.	2.2	X	X	X	X
Epigenetic determinism	Combination of a) *Covert genetic determinism* and b) the scientifically not validated assumption of the possibility of a voluntary influencing of one's own epigenome and the epigenome of future generations and the responsibility derived from this.	2.2		X	X	X
Genetic (data) exceptionalism	Ethical-legal requirement that genetic data should be given an exceptionally high level of protection.	2.3			X	X
Epigenetic (data) exceptionalism	Ethical-legal requirement that epigenetic data should be given an exceptionally high level of protection.	2.3				X

Areas of discourse (abbreviations): Scien.= Scientific discourse; P.-Scien. = Popular science texts, e.g., guidebooks; Soc. = Societal discourse; Eth. = Ethical discourse. The occurrence of the individual *-isms* in the respective discourse areas is hypothetical, especially for societal discourse. Observations are based on assessments of the secondary literature on the respective concepts.

ic determinism (2.2), genetic exceptionalism and epigenetic exceptionalism (2.3) (table 2).

We are aware that determinism, in particular, is a very strong term that suggests complete external determination.[9] We use this and the other -isms merely in reference to terms already introduced in ethical discourse, and do not wish to proclaim ourselves that humans are completely determined by their genes or epigenome.

In societal discourse, both ideas of genetic and epigenetic determinism are still present despite scientific findings that conflict with these concepts. Consequently, following an introduction to the various -isms, and in light of the new possibilities for intervening in both the genome and, in the future, perhaps also the epigenome of a human being, it may be asked: Can the procedures of genome and epigenome editing help to refute the assumption of genetic and epigenetic determinism or, on the contrary, do these new gene therapy procedures promote the notions of genetic and epigenetic determinism that are present in the current public discourse? This question is important for a critical reflection upon the -isms introduced here, and, thus, important for future research.

2.1 Genetic Essentialism and Strong Genetic Determinism

a) Concept

Genetic essentialism is based on the idea that the genotype completely determines the phenotype and the entire essence of a human being: "Genetic essentialism reduces the self to a molecular entity, equating human beings, in all their social, historical, and moral complexity, with their genes."[10] This implies that the human being as such is solely, or at least to a significant degree, determined by its genes. This concept stands disproved by science.[11]

Furthermore, just as questionable as genetic essentialism—and necessary precondition of it—is the concept of strong genetic determinism. David Resnik and Daniel Vorhaus define strong genetic determinism as the assumption that "gene G almost always leads to the development of trait T. (G increases the prob-

---

[9] D. B. Resnik and D. B. Vorhaus, "Genetic Modification and Genetic Determinism," *Philosophy, Ethics, and Humanities in Medicine* 1, no. 9, online publication, Jun. 26, 2006, DOI: 10.1186/1747-5341-1-9.

[10] D. Nelkin and M. Lindee, *The DNA Mystique: The Gene as a Cultural Icon* (New York: W. H. Freeman, 1995), 2.

[11] B. Tappeser and A.-K. Hoffmann, "Das überholte Paradigma der Gentechnik. Zum zentralen Dogma der Molekularbiologie fünfzig Jahre nach der Entdeckung der DNA-Struktur," in *Der kritische Agrarbericht 2004*, ed. AgrarBündnis e.V. (Hamm: ABL Verlag, 2004), 220–24, https://www.kritischer-agrarbericht.de/fileadmin/Daten-KAB/KAB-2004/Tappeser_Hoffmann.pdf; and Schuol, "Widerlegt die Epigenetik den Gendeterminismus?"

ability of T and the probability of T, given G, is 95% or greater)."[12] Although now refuted by recent findings in human genetics, this "one-gene-one-trait" relation was held to be valid for a long time even within science.[13] Therefore, it can be assumed that the ideas of strong genetic determinism as well as genetic essentialism are still present in society.[14]

b) Critique

Both positions (strong genetic determinism and genetic essentialism) are harshly rejected within the philosophy and ethics of science.[15] This is based not only upon the fact that they are scientifically refuted, but also on the belief that genetic essentialism has implications that are ethically worrisome. Ilan Dar-Nimrod and Steven Heine point out that the idea that a person would be determined entirely through his or her genes might result in selective discrimination of persons with certain characteristics and of their relatives, a discrimination that might not take place if these certain characteristics had a nongenetic cause: "research has shown that stronger genetic attributions for mental illness are associated with an increased desire for social distance from those with such illnesses ... and their kin."[16]

While genetic causality is perceived negatively in these situations, the contrary might also be the case. If one assumes that genes are natural, that what is natural is morally *good* (*naturalistic fallacy*), and if one furthermore assumes that genetic essentialism is true, that is, that human beings are entirely determined through their genes, then all human traits, characteristics, and behaviors are believed to be morally good. There is no room for critique. Instead, because of the deterministic understanding, every human behavior is perceived as legitimate. Only the artificial modification of the human genome would offer some room for critique, since a genetically modified genome would no longer be perceived as natural, and, according to the naturalistic fallacy, would no longer be considered morally good either, as noted parenthetically in the following quotation: "Furthermore, something may be more likely to be identified as natural to the extent that its existence is perceived to be predicated upon an underlying

---

[12] Resnik and Vorhaus, "Genetic Modification and Genetic Determinism" (see supra note 9).
[13] Tappeser and Hoffmann, "Das überholte Paradigma der Gentechnik" (see supra note 11); and Schuol, "Widerlegt die Epigenetik den Gendeterminismus?" (see supra note 7).
[14] Schuol, *Das regulierte Gen. Implikationen der Epigenetik für Biophilosophie und Bioethik* (see supra note 7).
[15] I. Dar-Nimrod and S. J. Heine, "Genetic Essentialism: On the Deceptive Determinism of DNA," *Philosophical Bulletin* 137, no. 5 (2011): 800–18, DOI: 10.1037/a0021860.
[16] Ibid., 808.

genetic predisposition (unless the genes themselves are the product of artificial manipulation as in the case of genetically-modified products)."[17]

One might wonder whether, according to this presupposition, every human being who, for instance, at the embryo stage had been genetically modified through germline interventions would be considered nonnatural and (by a naturalistic fallacy) *worse* morally speaking than a person whose genome had not been changed in that manner. Is the same to be assumed for a modification of the epigenome? Both conclusions might follow as a naturalistic fallacy from the position of strong genetic determinism and, as will be shown subsequently, from the additional assumption of epigenetic determinism. Therefore, genetic essentialism, strong genetic determinism, and epigenetic determinism are to be rejected, not only on scientific grounds but also on ethical grounds.

2.2 Covert Genetic Determinism and Epigenetic Determinism

a) Concept

Even *moderate* or *weaker* forms of genetic determinism, which merely assume that a gene sometimes leads to the expression of certain characteristics,[18] although scientifically correct, can become problematic from an ethical perspective if they are corroborated by further assumptions. These are the assumption that, by choosing their environmental conditions, individuals themselves can influence when a gene leads to the expression of particular characteristics, and the assumption that this particular epigenetic shaping of the genes can then also be passed on to future generations. Environmental conditions include nutrition (nutri-epigenetics). Following Miranda Waggoner and Tobias Uller (see supra note 7), we use the term epigenetic determinism to summarize these ideas. Epigenetic determinism is also based on assumptions that are partly unconfirmed scientifically. The assumption of transmission of acquired epigenetic modifications to future generations, albeit not validated, is based primarily on studies of the effects of malnutrition on subsequent generations.[19]

The concept of epigenetic determinism thus comprises the idea of genetic determinism, extended by the findings of epigenetics and further hypotheses concerning a perceived control of one's own epigenome and the epigenome of future generations and the responsibility derived from it. The latter in particular

---

[17] Ibid., 802.
[18] Resnik and Vorhaus, "Genetic Modification and Genetic Determinism" (see supra note 9).
[19] E. W. Tobi et al., "DNA Methylation Signatures Link Prenatal Famine Exposure to Growth and Metabolism," *Nature Communications* 5 (5592), Nov. 26, 2014, DOI: 10.1038/ncomms6592.

is problematic from a scientific point of view, since a direct control of one's own health and, in particular, the health of subsequent generations, mediated via the epigenome, cannot be, or at least has not yet been, proven in humans. Before coming back to this, however, some remarks concerning the assumption of genetic determinism extended by the findings of epigenetics are in order.

Sebastian Schuol describes covert genetic determinism as a disguised form of genetic determinism: "Der Phänotyp wird vom epigenetisch aktivierten Teil des Genoms determiniert" (The phenotype is determined by the epigenetically activated part of the genome).[20] This indicates that a gene does not directly result in the expression of a certain trait (phenotypic trait), as genetic determinism would claim, but rather that it only results in the expression of this trait when this gene is *epigenetically activated*. Epigenetic activation refers to a specific molecular configuration of DNA. For example, a gene is epigenetically activated if the DNA has a certain methylation state, since transcription of DNA (*reading*) is, in simple terms, possible only if the base cytosine (a component of DNA) is not methylated, that is, if no methyl group is attached to the cytosine in certain cytosine-rich parts of the genome, so-called CpG islands.[21] In accordance with the current understanding of epigenetics, expressed in covert genetic determinism, the genome continues to determine the phenotypic characteristics of a person.

Both Schuol, and Waggoner and Uller,[22] in their respective analyses of the influence of epigenetics findings on the concept of genetic determinism in science, popular science, and society, adopt a molecular genetics notion of epigenetics that includes, for example, DNA methylation. The two analyses draw a similar conclusion: it seems that in both popular and scientific discourse, the concept of epigenetics is invoked to refute genetic determinism, but genetic determinism persists in a covert form.

b) Critique

In the field of ethics, criticism is also leveled at the concept of covert genetic determinism.[23] It is correct from a scientific point of view that, as Schuol writes, *the phenotype is determined by the epigenetically activated part of the genome.* That is, whether a gene leads to the formation of a certain trait depends, among

---

[20] Schuol, "Widerlegt die Epigenetik den Gendeterminismus?" (see supra note 7), 53.
[21] C. W. Hanna and G. Kelsey, "The Specification of Imprints in Mammals," *Heredity* 113 (2014): 176–83, DOI: 10.1038/hdy.2014.54. This is where epigenome editing comes in, which aims to influence the transcription of certain genes by changing the epigenome, for example, the methylation state of DNA (see table 1).
[22] Waggoner and Uller, "Epigenetic Determinism in Science and Society" (see supra note 7).
[23] Schuol, *Das regulierte Gen. Implikationen der Epigenetik für Biophilosophie und Bioethik* (see supra note 7).

other things, on whether, simply put, the gene is epigenetically activated. We have described above the molecular genetic aspects of this. On one hand, however, covert genetic determinism is problematic if one assumes that humans are influenced only by their epigenetically activated genome and not, for example, also by their socialization. On the other hand, covert genetic determinism is also ethically problematic when it turns into epigenetic determinism. We define epigenetic determinism as follows:

> *Epigenetic determinism* is a combination of:
> (a) *Covert genetic determinism* and
> (b) the scientifically not validated assumption of the possibility of a voluntary influencing of one's own epigenome and the epigenome of future generations and the responsibility derived from this.

Presupposition (b) can be found in popular science texts, such as guidebooks or scientific media texts, as Schuol noted, and in this respect has an influence on public perceptions of epigenetics. This assumption of responsibility for one's own health, and the health of future generations, based on the possibility of changing the epigenome through a deliberate choice of environmental conditions, and thus influencing the *reading* of certain genes, whereby these changes in the epigenome can be stable over several generations, cannot be confirmed scientifically. On the contrary, there are even some reasons against it. For instance, some kind of epigenetic inheritance in humans is ruled out by the fact that the epigenome is almost completely reconfigured twice during the development of egg/sperm cells and embryos (so-called *epigenetic reprogramming*).[24] The scientifically unconfirmed assumption (b) is nevertheless sometimes defended in discourses on epigenetics.

Thus, the concept of epigenetic determinism serves as a descriptor of the current discussions on genetics and epigenetics. Since it is based on scientifically unproven premises, the conclusions regarding responsibility for one's own health, and the health of one's own children or later generations, are not justified and are ethically problematic. Epigenetic determinism can sometimes also be detected in ethics texts (see below, section 3.2). However, an essential prerequisite for a well-founded ethical debate is that it be based on the current state of science. The current state of science provides no evidence for the intergenerational heritability of acquired epigenetic changes in humans. Therefore, it is astonishing how long arguments about the responsibility for next generations persist and are repeated in the ethical discussion of epigenetics.

The goal of creating awareness for the concepts of covert genetic determinism and epigenetic determinism is to revisit those consequences that are ethi-

---

[24] Hanna and Kelsey, "The Specification of Imprints in Mammals" (see supra note 21).

cally problematic. Schuol draws attention to this problematic nature of attributions of responsibility in popular scientific discourses on epigenetics. In section 3, we will explain that precisely because of the deterministic conception of epigenetics, ethical discourses on epigenetics are analogous to discourses on genome editing.

2.3 Genetic Exceptionalism and Epigenetic Exceptionalism with Regard to Informational Self-Determination

a) Concept

Although we have characterized both strong genetic determinism and epigenetic determinism as problematic from a scientific and ethical perspective, there is some merit to the idea that genetic and perhaps epigenetic personal or population data should enjoy special legal protection.[25] This idea is also referred to as *genetic* or *epigenetic exceptionalism*, with genetic exceptionalism being the older and more widespread of the two concepts or ethical-legal postulates. Genetic exceptionalism is the claim for special protection of genetic data (for example, whole-genome sequencing data obtained in research or diagnostic genetic testing). This concept can be found in ethical debates but is sometimes also criticized. In what follows, we examine whether there is any justification for a critique of genetic exceptionalism. In addition, we consider the possibility of supplementing genetic exceptionalism by a requirement to provide special protection for epigenetic data as well, thus adding epigenetic exceptionalism to genetic exceptionalism.

b) Critique

Arguing against Genetic and Epigenetic (Data) Exceptionalism
The criticism of genetic essentialism is closely related to the critique in medical ethics of the concept of genetic exceptionalism in debates about the special treatment of genetic versus nongenetic medical information, especially with regard to a higher-ranking legal claim for protection of genetic data compared to nongenetic data. This is because the concept of genetic exceptionalism would be plausible if one assumed that persons with certain genetic characteristics suffer discrimination because other persons adopt the concept of genetic essentialism

---

[25] On ethical issues related to brain data, see F. Molnár-Gábor and A. Merk, "Spotlight. Die datenschutzrechtliche Bewertung von Neurodaten," in Fehse et al., *Fünfter Gentechnologiebericht*, 360–70; on big data and personalized medicine, see E. C. Winkler and B. Prainsack, "Big Data in der personalisierten Medizin—ethische Herausforderungen und Lösungsansätze," in Fehse et al., *Fünfter Gentechnologiebericht*, 371–400.

and therefore discriminate against individuals with certain genetic characteristics. This would mean that third parties assumed that only the invariable genetic characteristics (almost) completely determine the nature of these persons (genetic essentialism). In order to avoid discrimination based on this assumption, it would be necessary to provide special protection for genetic data compared to other medical or personal data against access by third parties.[26] Yet, since genetic essentialism in fact has proven to be false, arguing that genetic data should enjoy a higher level of protection than nongenetic data would in fact be scientifically implausible. This is because not only genetic but also epigenetic and other information about individuals and groups of individuals is highly informative—for example, with regard to sensitive characteristics of these individuals. Charles Dupras and Eline Bunnik offer numerous examples for this usefulness, including the re-identifiability of individuals on the basis of both their genetic and nongenetic data.[27] The authors explicitly oppose genetic exceptionalism, and instead advocate a "multi-omic contextualism." Within this contextualism approach, safeguarding different research data does not depend on which data type it belongs to. Instead, it is a matter of how sensitive the data are in each case, and how dire the consequences of data misuse would be.

In earlier versions of their contextualism model, Dupras and colleagues have already pointed out that the special protection claim of genetic data (genetic exceptionalism) must be complemented by a special protection claim of epigenetic data, as these are equally sensitive.[28] Dupras's and Bunnik's more recent contextualism model is also based primarily on an analysis of genetic and epigenetic data, yet Dupras and Bunnik[29] implicitly reject not only genetic but also epigenetic exceptionalism.[30] Their argument against these two concepts is that

---

[26] M. J. Green and J. R. Botkin, "'Genetic Exceptionalism' in Medicine: Clarifying the Differences between Genetic and Nongenetic Tests," *Annals of Internal Medicine* 138, no. 7 (2003): 571–75, DOI: 10.7326/0003-4819-138-7-200304010-00013.

[27] C. Dupras and E. M. Bunnik, "Toward a Framework for Assessing Privacy Risks in Multi-omic Research and Databases," *The American Journal of Bioethics* 21, no. 12 (2021): 46–64, DOI: 10.1080/15265161.2020.1863516.

[28] C. Dupras et al., "Epigenetic Discrimination: Emerging Applications of Epigenetics Pointing to the Limitations of Policies against Genetic Discrimination," *Frontiers in Genetics* 9 (2018), 202, DOI: 10.3389/fgene.2018.00202; and C. Dupras et al., "Selling Direct-to-Consumer Epigenetic Tests: Are We Ready?," *Nature Reviews Genetics* 21 (2020): 335–36, DOI: 10.1038/s41576-020-0215-2.

[29] Dupras and Bunnik, "Toward a Framework for Assessing Privacy Risks" (see supra note 26).

[30] K. Alex and E. C. Winkler, "Is Dupras' and Bunnik's Framework for Assessing Privacy Risks in Multi-omic Research and Databases Still Too Exceptionalist?," *The American Journal of Bioethics* 2, no. 12 (2021): 80–82, DOI: 10.1080/15265161.2021.1991039.

other types of data, depending on the context, have a similarly high sensitivity and therefore a similarly high demand for protection as genetic and epigenetic data.

Arguments in Favor of Genetic and Epigenetic Exceptionalism

The demand for genetic exceptionalism is initially supported by the entirely justified assumption—even without the need to advocate for strong genetic determinism—that genetic data have a particularly high informative value. On one hand, genetic data often allow predictive statements—for example, concerning the risk for the occurrence of a certain disease. On the other hand, they have an informative value that extends beyond the realm of the individual to genetically related family members. However, Dupras and Bunnik note that these two properties (predictivity and informative value with respect to third parties) could also apply to nongenetic data. As an example, they cite epigenetic variants shared by different members of a social community.[31] In addition, it could be that a combination of epigenetic and genetic data increases the risk of re-identifiability, which is why it should be considered to complement a genetic exceptionalism with an epigenetic exceptionalism.

Implications of Strong Genetic and Epigenetic Determinism for Genetic and Epigenetic Exceptionalism

Nanibaa' Garrison and colleagues point out that there are few proponents of genetic exceptionalism within ethical discourse at present.[32] However, the following argument supports the case for genetic exceptionalism: While it is true that genetic determinism has been scientifically disproven, ethics should not turn away from the subject too soon. For if the concept is spread in popular scientific discourse, and if many people continue to believe that our genes largely determine us, then they will act accordingly. As a result, this misperception could continue to cause people to be discriminated against. If so, ethics must continue to deal with the implications of these false assumptions.

So, to argue that genetic health care and research data are entitled to special protection, it is only necessary to assume that the notion of strong genetic determinism or genetic essentialism is prevalent in society—more precisely, that it prevails among third parties who might discriminate against individuals on the basis of their genetic characteristics. However, it is not a necessary (but possibly a sufficient) condition to be a proponent of the assumption of strong genetic de-

---

[31] Dupras and Bunnik, "Toward a Framework for Assessing Privacy Risks" (see supra note 26), 5.

[32] N. A. Garrison et al., "Genomic Contextualism: Shifting the Rhetoric of Genetic Exceptionalism," *The American Journal of Bioethics* 19, no. 1 (2019): 51–63, at 53, DOI: 10.1080/15265161.2018.1544304.

terminism or essentialism in order to support genetic exceptionalism. The same applies, moreover, to ethically problematic ideas about epigenetics. As long as the opinion prevails that, due to epigenetic controllability of gene regulation, individuals are to be held responsible for their own health, ethics must deal with the social consequences of this assumption. This would include the demand to place not only genetic but also epigenetic data under special protection in order to avoid discrimination on the basis of these data (epigenetic exceptionalism).

The aspect of heredity is also important here. While genetic determinism seems justified at least insofar as genetic information is indeed inherited, it appears that the assumption of heritability as part of epigenetic determinism serves a crucial role in the ethical discourse on epigenetics as well, yet it differentiates the significance of genetic and epigenetic information, and possibly underlines the exceptional claim to protection of genetic data (genetic exceptionalism).

However, calls for genetic and epigenetic exceptionalism would have to be accompanied by efforts to raise public awareness about the scientifically and ethically problematic assumptions of strong genetic and epigenetic determinism. This is because false assumptions regarding epigenetics lead to ethically problematic attributions of responsibility (epigenetic determinism). False assumptions regarding genetics (strong genetic determinism) can lead, for example, to a naturalistic fallacy that labels everything genetic as natural and everything natural as good, or they can result in discrimination against individuals with certain genetic traits. After all, without this critical understanding of the concepts examined here, it is possible that calls for genetic and epigenetic exceptionalism in relation to the handling of genetic and epigenetic data could reinforce the problematic assumptions of strong genetic and epigenetic determinism. Therefore, the present chapter aims to raise awareness of a critical approach to explicit and implicit -isms related to ideas about genetics, epigenetics, and gene technology.

3. Ethical Discourse about Epigenetics and Genome Editing—Similarities and Discrepancies in Key Aspects

3.1 Determinism

The deterministic understanding outlined in the previous section has the effect that debates on ethical aspects of genetics and epigenetics display strong parallels to the ethical discourse on the therapeutic use of genome editing in humans. The main parallel derives from the relevance of the reference to a possible genetic or (scientifically unverified) epigenetic inheritance and the responsibility derived from this for future generations.

In the ethical controversy on genome editing, we encounter divergent positions regarding the question of how the aspect of heritability of germline interventions should be judged ethically. There are positions which start from a moral imperative for research into therapeutic or even *enhancing*[33] applications of germline genome editing,[34] as opposed to positions that call for a moratorium with regard to research into genome editing on embryos.[35] Therapeutic modification of the genome is thus associated with high hopes of positive effects that last over several generations (for example, the hope of no longer passing on a genetically linked disease that has occurred frequently within a family in the past). However, fear of serious negative consequences that could also be passed on to multiple generations is also central to debates on genome editing. Part of the explanation for these extreme positions (imperative vs. moratorium) in the discourse on genome editing of embryos can be found in the special significance of intervening in the genome because of the assumption of genetic determinism.

3.2 Complexity within the Question and Dissolution of Boundaries

Another common feature of the discourses on genetics and genome editing as well as on epigenetics is the difficulty of evaluating these topics ethically. This difficulty arises from the complexity of the scientific premises, especially with regard to the dissolution of clear causal relationships between gene or genome, epigenome, and environment. There is ambiguity about what falls under the term "heredity" as a consequence of those boundary dissolutions. For example, Tim Lewens[36] and Stephan Guttinger[37] analyze genome editing from an ethical

---

[33] On the concept of an enhancing germline intervention, see Birnbacher, "Gentechnisches Enhancement" (see supra note 8).

[34] J. Savulescu et al., "The Moral Imperative to Continue Gene Editing Research on Human Embryos," *Protein Cell* 6, no. 7 (2015): 476–49, DOI 10.1007/s13238-015-0184-y.

[35] E. S. Lander et al., "Adopt a Moratorium on Heritable Genome Editing," *Nature* 567, no. 7747 (2019): 165–68, DOI: 10.1038/d41586-019-00726-5. Of the sixty-one position papers on genome editing surveyed by Carolyn Brokowski that appeared between 2015 and 2018, only 5 percent explicitly oppose such a moratorium: C. Brokowski, "Do CRISPR Germline Ethics Statements Cut It?," *The CRISPR Journal* 1, no. 2 (2018): 115–25, DOI: 10.1089/crispr.2017.0024.

[36] T. Lewens, "Blurring the Germline: Genome Editing and Transgenerational Epigenetic Inheritance," *Bioethics* 34, no. 1 (2020): 7–15, DOI: 10.1111/bioe.12606.

perspective with explicit reference to findings in epigenetics, and they derive the complexity of the question of an ethical analysis of genome editing from a postgenomic understanding of heredity.

However, the possibility to modify the genome or the epigenome by means of genetic engineering could already complicate concepts of genetic inheritance and epigenetic causation and dissolve previously existing boundaries, even if there is no indication of a connection between genetic and epigenetic causation. This is the case when the intervention in the genome or epigenome is described as an *artificial* alteration of *natural* genetic and epigenetic functional relationships. The ethical relevance of the difference between *naturalness* and *artificiality* in this context depends, among other things, on whether a naturalistic fallacy occurs (see 2.1). What has also been discussed in medical ethics is the question of whether an alteration of genetic information in the context of assisted reproductive technologies (ARTs) has an impact on the concept of genetic parenthood.[38] Given that genome editing might be used as an ART in the future[39] and that genetic information is altered in this process as well, Monika Piotrowska's question in the article "Why is an egg donor a genetic parent, but not a mitochondrial donor?"[40] could be complemented by the question whether genome and epigenome editing on embryos or fetuses also have consequences for the concept of genetic parenthood.

Dissolving the boundaries between genetic and nongenetic causation creates a complex baseline, both scientifically and ethically, for the analysis of epigenetics and genome editing. According to Sofia Falomir, this results in the need for the epigenetics discourse to also dissolve the boundaries of the disciplines in order to analyze epigenetics scientifically.[41] The same is true for discussions on genome editing, which, especially due to the notion of (covert) genetic determinism, must always be considered from multiple disciplinary perspectives at the

---

[37] S. Guttinger, "Editing the Reactive Genome: Towards a Postgenomic Ethics of Germline Editing," *Journal of Applied Philosophy* 37, no. 1 (2020): 58–72, DOI: 10.1111/japp.12367.

[38] M. Piotrowska, "Why Is an Egg Donor a Genetic Parent, but Not a Mitochondrial Donor?," *Cambridge Quarterly of Healthcare Ethics* 28, no. 3 (2019): 488–98, DOI: 10.1017/s0963180119000410.

[39] National Academy of Sciences et al., *Heritable Human Genome Editing: Consensus Study Report* (Washington, DC: National Academies Press, 2020).

[40] Mitochondria are cell organelles that are responsible for the energy supply of the cell. They are inherited from the mother's egg cell and contain their own DNA (mtDNA). In the case of certain diseases caused by nonfunctional mitochondria, ARTs can be used in various ways to ensure that the mitochondria are exchanged for those of a donor.

[41] S. Falomir, "Epigenetics and Metaphor: Language of Limits," *Technoethic Arts* 16, no. 3 (2018): 259–302, DOI: 10.1386/tear.16.3.295_1.

same time, so that deterministic notions can be scientifically tested and their ethical consequences highlighted. The need for an interdisciplinary approach is thus common to discourses on epigenetics as well as on genome editing.

3.3 Domains of Discourse on Epigenetics: Heritability, Responsibility, Justice

a) Heritability and Responsibility

In the ethical discourse on epigenetics, the question of responsibility is addressed. For example, a research report on epigenetics from the Berlin-Brandenburg Academy of Sciences and Humanities, cited at the beginning of this chapter, states: "Besondere Brisanz hat die Frage, in welchem Maß es eine epigenetische Verantwortung des Individuums für die Gestaltung der Lebensumstände nachfolgender Generationen gibt" (The question of the extent to which individuals have an epigenetic responsibility for shaping the living conditions of subsequent generations is particularly explosive).[42]

Schuol, in his ethical analysis of the popular scientific discourse on epigenetics, also points to the centrality of the question of responsibility:

> On the part of popular science guides ... three main topics are discussed. ... 1. the epochal change initiated by epigenetics and the replacement of geneticism, 2. the thereby promoted topic of lifestyle-related controllability of gene regulation, and 3. areas of responsibility resulting from this controllability. ...The statement that a *transgenerational responsibility* is connected with epigenetics was narrowed down: Several reasons speak against an epigenetic inheritance in humans.[43]

This is in line with the concept of epigenetic determinism described above. Schuol, as well as Jörn Walter and Anja Hümpel, draws attention to difficulties with the assumption of epigenetic determinism, as the latter is based on scien-

---

[42] J. Walter and A. Hümpel, eds., *Epigenetik. Implikationen für die Lebens und Geisteswissenschaften* (see supra note 6), 28.

[43] Schuol, *Das regulierte Gen. Implikationen der Epigenetik für Biophilosophie und Bioethik* (see supra note 7), 368–71, emphasis in original: "Auf Seiten populärwissenschaftlicher Ratgeber werden ... drei Hauptthemen diskutiert. ... 1. der durch die Epigenetik eingeleitete Epochenwandel und die Ablösung von einem Genfatalismus, 2. das dadurch beförderte Thema lebensstilbedingter Steuerbarkeit der Generegulation und 3. sich in Folge dieser Steuerbarkeit ergebende Verantwortungsbereiche. ... Die Aussage, dass mit der Epigenetik eine *transgenerationale Verantwortung* verbunden sei, wurde eingegrenzt: Gegen eine epigenetische Vererbung beim Menschen sprechen mehrere Gründe."

tific presuppositions that cannot be confirmed. Nevertheless, the assumption of a *lifestyle-related controllability of gene regulation*, which, as explained above, includes, for example, nutrition, coupled with the assumption of an *epigenetic inheritance*, can be found not only in popular science but also, as a consequence, within social discourse. But such an epigenetic determinism can also be identified within the ethical discourse on epigenetics.

As a result, ethical analyses of epigenetics are widely divergent. There are two basic approaches. Either it is assumed that epigenetic inheritance and responsibility for future generations do exist.[44] Or notions about an epigenetic foundation of intergenerational epigenetic responsibility are strongly rejected.[45] Only the latter, as shown above, corresponds to the current scientific state of the art. The assumption of epigenetic inheritance and responsibility for future generations is therefore invalid as long as it is not scientifically proven.

b) Justice

In epigenetics discourse, the aspect of responsibility for future generations resulting from the assumption of epigenetic determinism is also referred to as *intergenerational justice*. Since epigenetic determinism is based on the assumption that it is possible to influence the epigenome, and thus one's own health, through a conscious choice of environmental conditions, the epigenetics discourse calls for *environmental justice* (healthy environmental conditions for all). Supplemented by the demand for equitable access to health care, there is a triad: "environmental justice, intergenerational equity, and equitable access to healthcare."[46]

The aspect of environmental justice marks a central difference between the discourses on genome editing and on epigenetics. Here it becomes clear that discussions on epigenetics are more likely to be located in the field of public health ethics, whereas the debate on genome editing, although also partly carried out in this field with reference to distributive justice, predominantly adopts an approach based on the perspective of individual ethics. Thus, the three-part demand for environmental justice, intergenerational justice, and equitable access

---

[44] P. Bode, "Identität und Nichtidentität. Intergenerationale Gerechtigkeit als Gegenstand einer Ethik der Epigenetik," in Heil et al., *Epigenetik. Ethische, rechtliche und soziale Aspekte* (see supra note 7), 59–73.

[45] For example, Schuol, "Widerlegt die Epigenetik den Gendeterminismus?" (see supra note 7); and J. Y. Huang and N. B. King, "Epigenetics Changes Nothing: What a New Scientific Field Does and Does Not Mean for Ethics and Social Justice," *Public Health Ethics* 11, no. 11 (2018): 69–81, DOI: 10.1093/phe/phx013.

[46] C. Dupras and V. Ravitsky, "The Ambiguous Nature of Epigenetic Responsibility," *Journal of Medical Ethics* 42, no. 8 (2016): 534–41, at 538, DOI: 0.1136/medethics-2015-103295.

to health is to be understood primarily as a demand at the institutional level. Dupras and colleagues therefore attribute responsibility for one's own health and the health of future generations not to the individual but to the institutions of the state. "It would thus be unfair to blame the poor for being malnourished or living in toxic environments, factors that, through epigenetics, can negatively affect their own as well as their children's health."[47] It is important to point out once again that from a scientific point of view, the assumption of some kind of epigenetic inheritance in humans, which is reflected in this quotation, cannot be substantiated.

3.4 Domains of Discourse on Genome Editing: Safety, Consent, Future Generations

The demand for equitable access to promising gene therapy methods is also central to debates on genome editing.[48] In addition, the relevance of the aspect of inheritance in particular points to a further commonality with discourses on epigenetics. Debates on genome editing are predominantly concerned with ethical questions arising from germline interventions, and have from their very beginning focused on the responsibility for future generations.[49] The call for a moratorium on research into germline genome editing thus arises from concerns that the effects of intervening in the genome at the germline level (for example, on embryos) can be inherited by future generations.

a) Safety

Since the effects of genome editing with a therapeutic intention are not fully known in advance, a serious safety issue of germline genome editing is that any adverse effects can be passed on to countless downstream generations. For this reason, one necessary precondition for such an intervention is generally referred to as sufficient safety.[50] The following recommendation from U.S. and UK scientific societies on germline genome editing provides an example:

---

[47] C. Dupras et al., "Epigenetics and the Environment in Bioethics," *Bioethics* 28, no. 7 (2014): 327–34, at 333, DOI: 10.1111/j.1467-8519.2012.02007.x.

[48] I. van Dijke et al., "The Ethics of Clinical Applications of Germline Genome Modification: A Systematic Review of Reasons," *Human Reproduction* 33, no. 9 (2018): 1777–96, DOI: 10.1093/humrep/dey257.

[49] E. Agius and S. Busuttil, eds., *Germ-Line Intervention and Our Responsibilities to Future Generations* (Dordrecht: Spinger/Kluwer, 1998).

[50] S. Holm, "Let Us Assume That Gene Editing Is Safe: The Role of Safety Arguments in the Gene Editing Debate," *Cambridge Quarterly of Healthcare Ethics* 28, no. 1 (2019): 100–11, DOI: 10.1017/S0963180118000439.

Before any attempt to establish a pregnancy with an embryo that has undergone genome editing, preclinical evidence must demonstrate that heritable human genome editing (HHGE) can be performed with sufficiently high efficiency and precision to be clinically useful. For any initial uses of HHGE, preclinical evidence of safety and efficacy should be based on the study of a significant cohort of edited human embryos and should demonstrate that the process has the ability to generate and select, with high accuracy, suitable numbers of embryos that:
- have the intended edit(s) and no other modification at the target(s);
- lack additional variants introduced by the editing process at off-target sites—that is, the total number of new genomic variants should not differ significantly from that found in comparable unedited embryos;
- lack evidence of mosaicism introduced by the editing process;
- are of suitable clinical grade to establish a pregnancy; and
- have aneuploidy rates no higher than expected based on standard assisted reproductive technology procedures.[51]

b) Consent

In addition to safety, a particularly significant aspect in the ethical discourse on genome editing concerns the fact that, on one hand, a germline intervention is necessarily carried out without the consent of the person concerned, insofar as it is performed on embryos; embryos of course are not yet capable of giving consent. On the other hand, the intervention also has effects on potential offspring of these embryos due to its hereditary nature. These offspring also cannot consent to the intervention, since they do not yet exist. Thus: "issues of consent and threats to the autonomy of future generations are coming to the forefront of the debate."[52]

Linked to the problem of safety, the consent issue seems particularly relevant for genome editing on embryos. This is because it is seemingly impossible to resolve the problem of uncertainty about potentially serious negative consequences before the technique is first used on human embryos.[53]

That a medical intervention sometimes has to be carried out without the consent of the person concerned is a problem well known from other contexts—for example, in the treatment of children, unconscious persons, and other nonconsenting persons. In the debate on genome editing, however, the problem of consent is particularly central, since medical interventions on embryos and with

---

[51] National Academy of Sciences et al., *Heritable Human Genome Editing* (see supra note 38), 142, recommendation 5.
[52] R. L. Mintz et al., "Will CRISPR Germline Engineering Close the Door to an Open Future?," *Science and Engineering Ethics* 25, no. 5 (2019): 1409–23, DOI: 10.1007/s11948-018-0069-6.
[53] Guttinger, "Editing the Reactive Genome" (see supra note 36).

relevance for future generations are nontypical cases in which consent cannot be obtained. For nonconsenting persons, the following generally applies:

a) at the time of an intervention to which they cannot consent, they already exist;
b) they have representatives who can make a decision in their interest (in the case of children, these are often their parents);
c) the intervention they cannot consent to is associated with more predictable risks than a first clinical use of genome editing would be (aspect of safety, see above); and
d) their existence does not depend on the intervention itself.

These four conditions do not apply to embryos on which genome editing is performed, nor to their potential offspring, that is, to future generations. A heritable intervention in the genome of embryos or germ cells is therefore problematic even if sufficient safety could be ensured, since even then the other three of the consent-related aspects (a, b, and d) do not apply.

c) Effects on Embryos and Future Generations

Despite the centrality of the consent problem in the current discourse on genome editing, there is also criticism of what it means. This is because this position omits reference to how such consent could be obtained.[54] However, within debates on genome editing, the problem of heritability of germline interventions is also seen as problematic for reasons other than the inability of embryos and future generations to consent.

Depending on the moral status of the embryo, it might be impermissible to use the embryo for genome editing research and to discard it afterwards. However, even if the embryo is not discarded after genome editing but is transferred for pregnancy, an intervention in its genome may be problematic for ethical reasons. This is partly based on the right of the embryo and its potential offspring to an open future.[55] Linked to this is the problem of a negative influence on the relationship between the generations, whereby one generation influences the composition of the genome of another generation, which is to be judged negatively from an ethical point of view.[56]

---

[54] G. Cavaliere, "Genome Editing and Assisted Reproduction: Curing Embryos, Society or Prospective Parents?," *Medicine, Health Care, and Philosophy* 21, no. 2 (2018): 215–25, at 218, DOI: 10.1007/s11019-017-9793-y.

[55] Going back to Joel Feinberg's concept of a "right of the child to an open future," see in the genome editing discourse, for example, Mintz et al., "Will CRISPR Germline Engineering Close the Door to an Open Future?" (see supra note 51).

[56] This reasoning traces back to Jürgen Habermas, *Die Zukunft der menschlichen Natur. Auf dem Weg zu einer liberalen Eugenik?* (Frankfurt am Main: Suhrkamp, 2001). It can

The moral status of the embryo is relevant not only for debates about genome editing at the germline level, but also in relation to so-called prenatal diagnosis (PND) and preimplantation genetic diagnosis (PGD). In PGD, embryos are genetically examined, and those among them that are supposedly "healthy" are then selected and implanted with the aim of establishing a pregnancy. In the ethical discourse on genome editing, it is sometimes assumed that genome editing could be an alternative to PGD. Some works therefore compare PGD and genome editing and come to different conclusions regarding which of the two reproductive technologies would be ethically preferable.[57] However, this comparison may be obsolete. After all, reproductive use of genome editing without subsequent preimplantation genetic diagnosis and embryo selection seems to be out of the question for reasons of safety.[58] If one assumes that the moral status of the embryo prohibits the selection of embryos in the context of assisted reproductive medicine, then both PGD and genome editing would not be acceptable.

4. Conclusion and Outlook

In summary, ethical arguments relating to future generations and justice play a central role in the discourse on both epigenetics and genome editing. We began this article by analyzing and critically discussing the following concepts: genetic determinism, which is the basis of genetic essentialism; epigenetic determinism; and genetic and epigenetic exceptionalism. The discussion of the ethical discourse on epigenetics shows that the notion of epigenetic determinism can sometimes be found not only in popular scientific discourse but also in ethical discourse. Ethical debates on epigenetics, however, often distance themselves from this deterministic understanding. As a result, the focus of ethical discourse on epigenetics shifts from responsibility for one's own health and that of future generations to justice. What is meant here is justice, for example, with regard to access to healthy environmental conditions, regardless of whether these contribute to health with or without epigenomic mediation.

---

be seen in the debate comparing genome editing and preimplantation genetic diagnosis in C. Rehmann-Sutter, "Why Human Germline Editing Is More Problematic Than Selecting between Embryos: Ethically Considering Intergenerational Relationships," *The New Bioethics* 24, no. 1 (2018): 9–25, DOI: 10.1080/20502877.2018.1441669. See also D. Lanzerath, "Ethische Kriterien und Argumente im Wandel der Zeit," in Hucho et al., *Vierter Gentechnologiebericht* (see supra note 8), 103–28, at 121.

[57] Rehmann-Sutter, "Why Human Germline Editing Is More Problematic Than Selecting between Embryos" (see supra note 55).

[58] National Academy of Sciences et al., *Heritable Human Genome Editing* (see supra note 38).

An analysis of the discourse on genome editing reveals that it is primarily germline interventions that are being ethically scrutinized, and that the focus here is on the aspect of heredity. The question is whether this is accompanied by an implicit genetic determinism or even a genetic essentialism: the determinism could lie in the centrality of the aspect of heritability, since only genetic information is inherited. Does the aspect of heredity and the modification of the genome play a more decisive role in debates on genome editing than the problem of safety? Is the problem that embryos and their potential offspring cannot consent to germline interventions given such a high priority because these are genetic interventions?

Ethical criticism of germline genome editing (research) is sometimes based on arguing that safety risks are too high, and that to protect the embryo, (consumptive) research on human embryos which could minimize these safety risks should not be done. Alternatively, ethical criticism of germline genome editing (research) might be based on genetic determinism or genetic essentialism. This is the case if genome editing is rejected essentially because of the problem of heritability of genetic interventions on the germline level. This seems to imply at least a kind of weak genetic essentialism. This is because the distinctiveness of the disposition of one generation over another would, in this line of reasoning, be derived from the fact that it is a genetic disposition.[59] Following such argumentation, a fundamentally nongenetic influence on future generations would thus be relevant only if it were a matter of an influence on the genome mediated, for example, via the epigenome.[60]

Under such a presupposition of strong genetic determinism supplemented by epigenetic determinism, not only genome editing but also epigenome editing would be ethically relevant precisely because it, too, would have an influence on the genome. How this influence of genome editing, and epigenome editing is ethically evaluated in each case therefore depends initially on whether the assumptions of genetic and epigenetic determinism are advocated. These assumptions are increasingly viewed critically in ethical discourse because they cannot be confirmed scientifically. In popular scientific debates in particular, however, they seem to persist, which ultimately also influences the public discussion. Since a broad public discussion is required especially for genome editing, a reflective handling of the different -isms analyzed in this chapter is central.

---

[59] We thank Christiane Woopen for a critical discussion of this aspect.
[60] Guttinger, "Editing the Reactive Genome" (see supra note 63), 67.

The Impact of Advances in Surgical Techniques and Quality-of-Life Considerations on Ethical Decision-Making and Education in Neurosurgery

Andreas Unterberg and Pavlina Lenga

Introduction

Progress in medicine has been enormous in the past twenty years, although some of this progress has not been recognized in full detail by the public. The treatment of widespread diseases such as arterial hypertension, diabetes, cardiac arrhythmia, and degenerative skeletal disease with guideline-based approaches has improved drastically, and oncological treatment has incorporated the use of novel chemotherapeutic and antibody-based strategies. Pediatricians can now cure rare cerebral defects with the aid of gene therapy, and the introduction of minimally invasive technologies has led to huge improvements in surgery. These advances are obvious, and they also account for the slowly but steadily increasing average life expectancy with a good or acceptable quality of life. All of this progress is very positive, and it is welcomed from all sides.

On the other hand, this undeniable progress does not come without enormous costs and consumption of available resources. Modern and future-oriented strategies in medicine can no longer be funded and paid for in many countries. As a result, many industrialized countries have opted for a responsible consideration of economic factors when using modern therapeutic procedures. However, concerns have been raised that medicine is becoming economized as a result of this development.

Only recently, a thesis paper of the German Medical Association requested a change of strategy, because an economic approach to the practice of medicine has become an extreme burden.[1] Without a doubt, it is essential to be thrifty with available resources of a solidarity-based health-care system. However, wrong incentives have been identified as a relevant problem in the past two de-

---

[1] Ärzteblatt, D.Ä.G., Redaktion Deutsches, "Thesen zur Ökonomisierung der ärztlichen Berufstätigkeit," *Deutsches Ärzteblatt* 119, no. 39 (2022), https://www.aerzteblatt.de/archiv/227779/Thesen-zur-Oekonomisierung-der-aerztlichen-Berufstaetigkeit.

cades. Very often, especially in surgical disciplines and comparable to the manufacturing industry, criteria such as frictionless processes, speed, and efficiency are encouraged. The economization of medical practice in surgical disciplines is associated with a concentration on high-profit procedures and increased case numbers, and, moreover, profit maximization is enabled through quantitative growth and increased time efficiency. Certainly, these issues were called to public attention through the so-called DRG (Systems Diagnosis Related Groups). The medical ethicist Giovanni Maio, at Freiburg, emphasized that "too little is taken into consideration that qualified medical practice is reflected by efforts to find a solution tailored to the specific situation of a patient rather than by a rigid adherence to rules."[2]

What exactly represents the improvement of quality in the treatment of surgical patients in particular? First, an implementation of guidelines that have been developed in a stepwise manner into clinical practice leads to a more standardized treatment. The next important issue to emphasize is that surgical training should be curricula-oriented to pass along guidelines and standards of (surgical) treatment in a comprehensive manner. Furthermore, a trend toward subspecialization in medicine indicates that operations are performed by particularly qualified surgeons in high-volume hospitals.

Not least, but rather first and foremost, the goal of surgical treatment is the promotion of an individual doctor-patient relationship, particularly in surgery. Surgical disciplines are not "contractual repair workshops" that carry out mechanical corrections, but they should be characterized by empathy, individualized patient education, and a patient-tailored treatment. Regrettably, it has become difficult to maintain a surgeon-patient relationship that incorporates all these principles. We would do well to remind ourselves of the ethical principles of medicine. The advent of new surgical techniques, especially in the neurosurgical field, has raised several ethical tensions in medicine. Therefore, the goal of this essay is to discuss these developments from an ethical point of view and to focus on quality-of-life issues as a way of proposing some guidelines.

Advances in Surgical Techniques

Surgery, like all other fields of medicine, comprises two elements: science and art. The art component relates to applied practice, surgical competencies, craftsmanship, and social behaviors. The scientific aspects of surgery include knowledge, information, critical thinking, reasoning, and analytical skills. The French

---

[2] Ärzteblatt, D.Ä.G., Redaktion Deutsches, "Ökonomisierung der Medizin: Sinnentleerung ärztlichen Tuns," *Deutsches Ärzteblatt* 119, no. 39 (2022), https://www.aerzteblatt.de/archiv/227769/Oekonomisierung-der-Medizin-Sinnentleerung-aerztlichen-Tuns.

neurosurgeon Anne-Laure Boch stated, "Modern surgery is the place where science became technoscience, the place where knowledge became power."[3] Science and technology are linked and grow together. Science and technology in medicine ensure that surgery achieves the desired efficacy, since medicine aims to be efficacious. One might wonder how efficacy can be interpreted, especially from the patient's perspective. Efficacy is equal to healing, albeit "healing" might be utopic since, even in the era of modern medicine, it cannot be achieved for all existing pathologies. For example, in neurosurgery, glioblastoma represents the most aggressive primary tumor in adults, with an average life expectancy despite maximal therapy (surgery, chemotherapy, and radiation) of no more than 17.8 to 23.5 months.[4] Even with advances in surgical techniques, including the introduction and use of navigation systems now routinely found in surgical theaters, such tumors, cannot be removed completely by surgery. In the 1990 s, minimally invasive approaches became possible as a result of the development of video camera systems and monitors. Since then, further advances, including robotic, natural orifice transluminal endoscopic, and endoluminal surgical techniques, have been introduced; hence, a process that integrates the biological, physical, and information sciences into medicine has been taking place.

Where Will Future Technological Developments Lead?

Technology-driven development has changed the standard approach in surgery for treatment and diagnosis and has led to a change in the spectrum of surgical diseases. Surgeons' basic skills have been replaced by emerging technologies. Besides technological advancements and innovation, an immense increase in knowledge and information has led to another challenge in surgical practice—the sub- or superspecialization. This challenge is inevitable in academia—hence, carrying the risk of merely creating a technician. Therefore, one might wonder where these technological achievements lead. What impact do they have on surgeons and patients? Can a surgeon be biased and driven by financial gains when proposing or approving a therapy? These and other questions need to be addressed and answered. Notwithstanding the various technological developments, it should always be remembered that the patient and respective benefi-

---

[3] Diana Cardenas, "Surgical Ethics: A Framework for Surgeons, Patients, and Society," *Revista do Colégio Brasileiro de Cirurgiões* 47, no. 7 (2020), https://doi.org/10.1590/0100-6991e-20202519.

[4] Aaron C. Tan et al., "Management of Glioblastoma: State of the Art and Future Directions," *CA: A Cancer Journal for Clinicians* 70 (2020): 299–312, https://doi.org/10.3322/caac.21613.

cial therapies remain the core mission of every physician, and even more so of surgeons.

Impacts of Advances in Surgical Techniques

Impact on Patients

Surgeons have technical capabilities (*techne*), scientific knowledge (*episteme*), and judgment capacity (*phronesis*) to propose a "rescue plan" to their patients. Patients often ask for the latest technologies, such as robotics and innovative surgeries, which might not be suitable or even possible, depending on the individual case.

Impact on Neurosurgeons

Personal experience and knowledge are important sources to guide surgical decision-making. However, some conflicts of interest (COI) are inevitably present and could influence decisions regarding procedures and the use of devices. The goal of medical devices is to improve outcomes of neurosurgical patients. Nevertheless, they should be used ethically and always to benefit the patient's therapy. Physicians and surgeons could be influenced by direct and indirect incentives. Direct incentives include financial ties with industry, which can lead to using particular devices for financial gains, and incentives to publish novel techniques to improve academic standing. Indirect incentives, including personal relationships with colleagues and industry representatives, could unduly influence decisions regarding selection of medical devices. Novel approaches can allow surgeons to improve their financial compensation, expand their referral volume, increase their productivity, and improve their reputation. However, the following sentence describes the surgeon's mission: "A surgeon must first gather all the facts about a patient's care by examining multiple dimensions of the patient's life, health, and desires."[5]

Impact on Neurosurgical Trainees (Residents)

One paramount aspect of ethical decision-making is education at the trainee level. This should promote ethical decision making and professionalism based on human values. Furthermore, personal development in a socially and ethically

---

[5] Cardenas, "Surgical Ethics."

responsible manner should be a major goal of neurosurgical residency or education. If young neurosurgeons receive such education during the early stages of their training, they can be better prepared for ethical decisions, particularly when they involve applying new technologies in a surgical environment. They should be able to recognize medical industrialization and economic pressure. It is critical to develop a model of collective deliberation that can help understand ethical problems as they arise. Young neurosurgeons should learn that medicine or surgery should be done ethically, even when applying modern technologies. The professionalism required from every trainee consists of three important factors: (1) the exclusive right to practice in a defined area of endeavor; (2) the right to professional autonomy; and (3) the duty to put the patient's interests ahead of one's own.

Impact on Society

Advances in surgical techniques and the widespread use of medical devices have substantially impacted society. The question is, *what does society expect?*

Justice is generally interpreted as fair, equitable, and appropriate treatment of persons. Of the several categories of justice, the one that is most pertinent to clinical ethics is distributive justice. Distributive justice refers to the fair, equitable, and appropriate distribution of health-care resources determined by justified norms that structure the terms of social cooperation. Valid principles of distributive justice could be an equal share according to need, according to effort, according to contribution, according to merit, and according to free-market exchanges. It is easy to see the difficulty in choosing, balancing, and refining these principles to form a coherent and workable solution to distribute medical resources. A few examples of issues of distributive justice encountered in hospital practice need to be mentioned. These include allotment of scarce resources (equipment, tests, medications, organ transplants) and care of patients without health-care insurance coverage. Difficult as it may be, and despite the many constraining forces, physicians must accept the requirement of fairness.

Impact on Decision-Making

Shared decision-making (SDM) is a process in which clinicians and patients collaborate to decide on the best treatment for a condition. SDM combines clinical expertise and evidence with the patient's experiences and preferences. Three essential components for effective SDM should be considered: (1) provision of reliable, evidence-based information that outlines treatment options, outcomes, and uncertainties and risks; (2) decision-support counseling aimed at clarifying options and preferences; and (3) a system for recording, communicating, and implementing the patient's preferences. The key to a right and ethical SDM process is *patient-centered treatment*.

Sociological Considerations

The effect of technological development and innovation on societies should be discussed, as access to surgical innovations and new technologies is generally limited to more highly developed countries or wealthier segments of the population within such countries. For example, the deployment of navigation systems or fiber tracking technologies in neurosurgery has enabled surgical removal of tumors that previously were considered inoperable. However, such tumors are still not amenable to surgery in developing countries, since the necessary tools are unavailable because of excessively high costs. Such differences have led to disparities in surgical care among nations. Besides innovation and technological development, market-based health reforms have led to the abandonment or loss of some professional values in medical practice at the expense of shifting the humanitarian approach to a business enterprise. Surgery is one of the fields of medical practice most affected by these changes.

The medical-device industry plays a paramount role in promoting innovations in neurosurgery by helping to fund and facilitate research, resulting in conflicts of interest (COI). Neurosurgeons are involved in this industry and help to develop new devices. Neurosurgeons provide critical insights into new technological developments, while the financial compensations reward the risk and help stimulate neurosurgeons to continue innovating. However, problems might arise if the business interests of a particular company impact clinical decision-making and patient care by neurosurgeons with COI.

Three factors should be considered, even among neurosurgeons without COIs: (1) improvement in financial outcomes; (2) publication of scientific results; and (3) gain of social status. All three factors can affect clinical decision-making and subsequent patient care. While these are important to the success and advancement of neurosurgery, the COIs that naturally develop during such innovative pursuits must be always be reported to ensure the protection of patients' safety. It is also critical to remember that relationships between industry and neurosurgeons can benefit patients by giving them access to cutting-edge treatments that bring hope. These relationships also provide physicians with new knowledge and a better understanding of the neurosurgical field. However, surgeons must be aware of their ethical obligation to act in the best interests of their patients and take an oath to uphold such ethical standards. The goal of every surgery is to achieve the best outcome and preserve or improve the patient's quality of life (QoL).

Quality of Life

Neurosurgical outcomes are measured by various factors, including quality of life (QoL), invasiveness of the surgery, and recovery time. All of these are essential components of complex surgical decision-making. However, how can surgical outcomes be measured? How can we evaluate whether surgery helped or improved the patient's condition? Issues related to QoL are widely discussed in this context, but what does this term mean?

One might argue that QoL means anything that makes life proceed optimally. QoL determines what benefits patients, their autonomous choices, their best interest, and the medical standard of care. Disease-specific symptoms, general health perception, somatic discomfort, social behaviors, role functioning, cognitive functioning, and psychological well-being are components of QoL that often guide clinical decision-making. These are the principles of QoL, which have been described by Monika Bulllinger and Julia Quitmann.[6] Here it is important to highlight those components, such as baseline functionality, lifestyle and dependency, expected time of recovery, and potential deficits resulting from the surgical approach. They should definitely be considered when trying to define or predict postoperative QoL.

QoL in the field of neurosurgery mainly depends on patient outcomes after surgery. Different scales have been developed to evaluate the QoL, depending on the location of the pathology (for example, intracranial or spinal). It is difficult to study symptoms that could have many potential contributing etiologies; therefore, better research models are needed to understand the symptom burden and contributors to decreased QoL and to develop targeted interventions to counter these. The major drawback of questionnaires examining QoL is assuredly the extended length or complexity of questions, which often results in noncompliance. Keeping it simple is the key to determining the quality of life!

Neuro-Oncology and Quality of Life

The increasing consideration being given to assessing patients' quality of life in contemporary neurosurgical clinical studies can be attributed to several factors, including technological advances with escalating costs, the lack of a clear benefit in terms of length of survival (a traditional outcome measure) in several recent clinical trials of different treatment modalities, and the obvious need to rationalize the practice of neurosurgery by adopting an evidence-based approach. The current emphasis on neuro-oncological patients' subjective experiences, sat-

---

[6] Monika Bullinger and Julia Quitmann, "Quality of Life as Patient-Reported Outcomes: Principles of Assessment," *Dialogues in Clinical Neuroscience* 16 (2014): 137–45.

isfaction, and preferences as the goal of health-care delivery also warranted development and psychometric validation of QoL instruments to assess these experiences and preferences. Three important aspects of QoL in patients with brain tumors were proposed by Raymond Liu and colleagues.[7] These aspects are patients, tumors, and treatment factors, all of which should be taken into account when treating patients with such complex pathologies.

Patient factors. Studies focusing on comorbidities and demographics of patients with brain tumors and their effects on QoL are lacking. However, patient comorbidities are important in determining the extent of surgery, since long operating times might contribute to high rates of complication or mortality in older patients with poor baseline health.

Tumor factors. Tumor location and laterality have been shown to correlate with several specific symptoms in some studies but not in others. Patients with tumors in the left hemisphere might have greater communication problems than those with tumors in the right hemisphere, even before treatment is initiated; therefore, the reliability of conclusions about laterality based on the symptoms and QoL is sometimes questionable. Cognitive function could also be related to tumor laterality. For example, left-hemisphere tumors have been associated with lower verbal test scores, whereas right-hemisphere lesions have been associated with lower facial-recognition test scores. Furthermore, tumors in eloquent cortex areas, including those associated with the cranial nerves, motor function, the visual system, and language, might be damaged by surgical resection. With the advent of new imaging tools, such as the delineation of brain fibers, known as fiber tracking, neurosurgeons can prepare their steps preoperatively and intraoperatively so that complications, such as new neurological deficits, are diminished. Nevertheless, such high-risk surgeries are potentially linked to severe complications; hence, postoperative QoL might be severely impaired.

Treatment factors. Treatment factors affecting the overall QoL of patients with brain tumors include surgery, radiation, chemotherapy, and associated medications. The relationships between QoL and these treatments have been studied, although such studies lacked adequate power and control populations. Radiation therapy might adversely affect the QoL of patients with brain tumors, leading to increased fatigue in the short term and contributing to cognitive dysfunction in the long term. Patients receiving chemotherapy might present symptoms such as vomiting, anorexia, constipation, and decreased social functioning.

---

[7] Raymond Liu et al., "Quality of Life in Adults with Brain Tumors: Current Knowledge and Future Directions," *Neuro-Oncology* 11 (2009): 330–39, https://doi.org/10.1215/15228517-2008-093.

Spinal Disorders and Quality of Life

Spinal disorders, especially lower back pain, affect many people and have a negative impact on their work capacity and overall well-being. Coupled with escalating health-care costs, lower back pain frequently results in significant impairment of physical and psychological health and a decline in the performance of social responsibilities at work and at home.[8] From 2005 to 2014, for instance, the overall prevalence of chronic lower back pain increased by 162 percent among females aged twenty-one to thirty-four years, and 320 percent among males aged forty-five to fifty-four years.[9] Changes in the demands of psychosocial and physical work have also been attributed to these increases in prevalence. Various scales have been proposed to evaluate low back pain and related postoperative outcomes.

Several aspects should be considered. Lower back pain is a major global health problem that affects both young and older patients.[10] Considering the range of spinal pathologies, young patients are mainly affected by acute-onset low back pain due to disc herniation, whereas older patients are affected by chronic low back pain due to degenerative alterations of their spine. However, such a distinction cannot be evaluated through the various questionnaires or scales that evaluate the patients' QoL. It is imperative to develop scales that consider various age groups and their unique needs to better evaluate the patients' presurgical condition and facilitate measuring postoperative improvements or deteriorations.

---

[8] Laxmaiah Manchikanti et al., "Epidemiology of Low Back Pain in Adults," *Neuromodulation Technology at the Neural Interface* 17 (2014): 3–10, https://doi.org/10.1111/ner.12018.

[9] Ibid.

[10] Jetan H. Badhiwala et al., "Comparison of the Inpatient Complications and Health Care Costs of Anterior versus Posterior Cervical Decompression and Fusion in Patients with Multilevel Degenerative Cervical Myelopathy: A Retrospective Propensity Score–Matched Analysis," *World Neurosurgery* 134 (2020): e112–e119, https://doi.org/10.1016/j.wneu.2019.09.132/; Michael G. Fehlings et al., "The Aging of the Global Population: The Changing Epidemiology of Disease and Spinal Disorders," *Neurosurgery* 77 Suppl. 4 (2015): S1–5, https://doi.org/10.1227/NEU.0000000000000953; and Michael G. Fehlings and Babak Arvin, "Surgical Management of Cervical Degenerative Disease: The Evidence Related to Indications, Impact, and Outcome," *Journal of Neurosurgery: Spine* 11 (2009): 97–100, https://doi.org/10.3171/2009.5.SPINE09210.

Decision-Making

Every surgeon is confronted with the question of how to optimally treat patients. This question presents three major issues:
- Is treatment possible? If so, how to treat?
- Why treat?
- When should treatment be stopped?

In answering these questions, four principles should be respected during the decision-making process, particularly if the surgeons are confronted with applying new technologies with questionable patient outcomes.[11] These principles include respect for the patient's autonomy (including informed consent), beneficence, nonmaleficence, and justice. These four principles guide the evaluation and interpretation of ethical issues in patient care. They are accepted as the basis for ethical decisions in medicine and surgery. Notably, they should not be seen as a checklist of actions informing physicians about the appropriate approach to any situation, but rather as a framework of virtues or values relevant to an ethical debate. Let us take a closer look at these four principles.

Respect for the Patient's Autonomy

Patients should be treated as autonomous persons. This means recognizing the individual's capacity for self-determination and ability to make independent decisions and authentic choices based on personal values and beliefs.
- Autonomy can be exercised only after obtaining full and appropriate information and understanding the information.
- Therefore, patients must be adequately informed about the benefits and risks of the proposed surgical treatment.
- Informed consent plays a significant role in the patient-surgeon relationship. The surgeon's final step in the information process is obtaining informed consent from patients before scheduled surgery. Providing informed consent is an important decision the patient must make freely and independently. The legal principle of informed consent for surgery emphasizes that the patient is an independent adult with the capacity and competence to authorize a procedure that would affect their body and mind. Therefore, any operation that may infringe upon this principle is illegal and ethically unacceptable.

---

[11] Cardenas, "Surgical Ethics."

Beneficence

The principle of beneficence imposes an obligation on the surgeon to act with the intention of doing good for the patient. Surgeons must comply with their professional obligations and standards to provide appropriate surgical interventions in response to medical indications and follow the consent provided by the patient.

Nonmaleficence

The principle of nonmaleficence stipulates the obligation not to inflict harm on others. Surgery should minimize all possible harm. To achieve this goal, surgeons must assess the nature and scope of all relevant risks and benefits.

Justice

The principle of justice addresses the need to provide all individuals with equal access to health care. Limited resources, including the availability of surgeons, other health personnel, and caregivers devoted to their patients, must be evenly distributed to benefit all patients. Resources should be distributed fairly without discrimination.

When Should Treatment Be Stopped?

The social commitment and ethical duty of the physician is to sustain life and relieve suffering. Where the performance of one duty conflicts with the other, preferences of the individual patient should always and in every manner prevail. The principle of patient autonomy requires that physicians respect the decision to forgo life-sustaining treatment of a patient who possesses decision-making capacity. In some circumstances, treatments might be no longer of benefit, while in others the patient or family no longer wants them. The physician plays an essential role in clarifying the goals of medical treatment, defining the care plan, initiating discussions about life-sustaining therapy, educating patients and families, helping them deliberate, making recommendations, and implementing the treatment plan. Communication might be the key tool. It should be clarified that when inevitable death is imminent, it is legitimate to refuse or limit forms of treatment that would only secure a precarious and burdensome prolongation of life, for as long as basic humane, compassionate care is not interrupted. Agreement to a Do Not Resuscitate (DNR) status does not preclude supportive measures that keep patients free from pain and suffering as much as possible. Clinical practice on withdrawing or withholding treatment should be based on a sufficient understanding of medical, ethical, cultural, and religious issues. Care options should be discussed with a view toward illness status and patient and family preferences, beliefs, values, and cultures. The process of shared decision-making among the patient, the family, and clinicians should continue as therapeutic goals evolve and change.

Examples from the Neurosurgical Field

Glioblastoma

Glioblastoma is the most aggressive brain tumor, associated with a poor survival of eighteen to twenty-four months with maximal therapy (surgery, chemotherapy, and radiation). Unsurprisingly, the postdiagnosis and pretreatment level of QoL in patients with glioma is significantly lower than that in healthy controls. Patients with glioma experience general cancer-related symptoms, such as fatigue, anxiety, and depression, and disease-specific symptoms, including seizures, cognitive deficits, motor dysfunction, and symptoms caused by elevated intracranial pressure, all of which might impair the QoL.

Glioma surgery aims to resect as much tumor tissue as possible. The intent is to alleviate symptoms and prolong survival while minimizing operation-related complications. Tumor resection could improve the QoL by alleviating the neurological symptoms and improving cognitive functioning as consequences of tumor mass reduction. Surgery might also damage the normal surrounding tissue and cause (mostly transient) neurological and cognitive deficits, thereby decreasing the QoL.

A nonrandomized prospective study of patients with high grade glioma (HGG) found a significant association between the extent of tumor resection and QoL.[12] Patients who underwent gross total or subtotal tumor resection were more likely to have an improved QoL than those who underwent biopsy only. These results should be interpreted with caution because of the bias introduced by patient selection based on tumor size and location and the patient's performance status.[13] In a low percentage, there is also long-term survival, in which QoL is affected in other manners. The physical improvements observed in long-term survivors during the first months after surgery could be attributed to recuperation after surgery and radiotherapy; however, this factor cannot fully explain

---

[12] Linda Dirven et al., "Health-Related Quality of Life in High-Grade Glioma Patients," *Chinese Journal of Cancer* 33 (2014): 40–45, https://doi.org/10.5732/cjc.013.10214.

[13] Ibid.

the subsequent improvements in the later stages of the disease. Although confronted with a brain tumor that carries a poor prognosis, long-term survivors complained less about future uncertainty. This attitude could be because the patients realized at that time that they were functioning relatively well after surgery and radiotherapy (known as the "survivorship" feeling).[14]

A very important aspect of therapy in the case of recurrent glioblastoma is to weigh risk and benefits of a second surgery, since survival might be prolonged by only a couple of months. A recent meta-analysis of 1,906 patients found that the survival time of patients who underwent reoperations for recurrences (n = 709) was longer than that of patients who received only conservative management after the first operation.[15] The reoperation results are thought to be better in more recent studies owing to advances in operating techniques and patient selection.[16] A retrospective study of 121 patients—30 percent of whom qualified for reoperation—found that the mean survival in the reoperated group was 10.5 months longer than for patients who were not reoperated on.[17] At this point in time, we cannot yet reliably predict who is most likely to benefit from a second surgery. The development of probabilistic models could support treatment decision-making. The scoring systems proposed to date, however, have typically been developed based on small patient cohorts (approximately one hundred), retrospectively analyzing data sets of patients who underwent a second surgery, disregarding the outcomes of those who did not. The factors in these models include age, Karnofsky performance index PS, and tumor volume.[18] It is assumed that surgery was appropriate only if the expected extent of resection was greater than 90 percent.[19] The RESURGE trial inclusion criteria targeted patients eligible for maximum resection, in whom complete resection of the contrast-enhanced tumor was considered feasible, and no eloquent cortex

---

[14] Ingeborg Bosma et al., "Health-Related Quality of Life of Long-Term High-Grade Glioma Survivors," *Neuro-Oncology* 11 (2009): 51–58, https://doi.org/10.1215/15228517-2008-049.

[15] Victor M. Lu et al., "The Survival Effect of Repeat Surgery at Glioblastoma Recurrence and Its Trend: A Systematic Review and Meta-Analysis," *World Neurosurgery* 115 (2018): 453–59.e3, https://doi.org/10.1016/j.wneu.2018.04.016

[16] Ibid.

[17] Juan Delgado-Fernandez et al., "Usefulness of Reintervention in Recurrent Glioblastoma: An Indispensable Weapon for Increasing Survival," *World Neurosurgery* 108 (2017): 610–17, https://doi.org/10.1016/j.wneu.2017.09.062.

[18] Paul M. Brennan et al., "Second Surgery for Progressive Glioblastoma: A Multi-Centre Questionnaire and Cohort-Based Review of Clinical Decision-Making and Patient Outcomes in Current Practice," *Journal of Neurooncology* (2021): 153 (2021), 99–107, https://doi.org/10.1007/s11060-021-03748-0.

[19] Ibid.

areas were involved.[20] Regardless of the surgical goals, the maintenance or improvement of the patient's QoL is of paramount importance; this needs to be discussed with the patients. Success in maintaining and maximizing the QoL depends, at least in part, on the patients' performance status.

Benign Brain Tumors

Special attention should be paid regarding the course of benign tumors. Surgical resection of tumor entities, such as benign craniopharyngiomas, might also lead to worsened QoL. They are rare benign tumors of the sellar and/or parasellar regions, varying in size and composition, and include cystic and solid parts. Based on the current literature, approximately 95 percent of all craniopharyngiomas show suprasellar extension, 20–41 percent show infrasellar growth, and 53–75 percent show both. Visual impairment is one of the main symptoms in patients with craniopharyngioma, both before and after surgery. It is manifested as impaired visual acuity, visual field deficits, or both. The existing literature disagrees on the neuropsychological outcomes after surgical removal of craniopharyngiomas. Major issues with these studies include small samples and the lack of "good" and "poor" neuropsychological outcome definitions. Therefore, comparisons between studies are limited. Klaus Zweckberger and colleagues reported, based on a prospective study, that patients with skull base meningiomas profited from surgical resection, showing significant improvements in neuropsychological outcomes and QoL.[21] On the other hand, Henrik Giese and colleagues detected a higher rate of postoperative neuropsychological impairment in attention, executive function, cognitive speed, working memory, and verbal memory in craniopharyngioma patients compared to the "normal" population.[22] Furthermore, impaired QoL in at least one dimension of the SF-36 questionnaire was detected in 75 percent of the patients. Therefore, one might argue that surgery should be considered carefully in the case of benign tumors, since patients can be negatively affected.[23]

Of note, the current aim of surgery for lesions within the pineal region is to obtain a histological diagnosis that can facilitate the planning of further treat-

---

[20] Ibid.

[21] Klaus Zweckberger et al., "Prospective Analysis of Neuropsychological Deficits Following Resection of Benign Skull Base Meningiomas," *Journal of Neurosurgery* 127 (2017): 1242–48, https://doi.org/10.3171/2016.10.JNS161936.

[22] Henrik Giese et al., "Neurological and Neuropsychological Outcome after Resection of Craniopharyngiomas," *Journal of Neurosurgery* 132 (2019): 1425–34, https://doi.org/10.3171/2018.10.JNS181557.

[23] Ibid.

ments and remove the lesion. Stepan Fedorko and colleagues found that surgical treatment of tumors in the pineal region improved the neurological status, decreased disability in most cases, and significantly increased the patients' QoL.[24] Furthermore, Fedorko and colleagues showed that radical tumor resection or cyst removal decreased the need for further surgical procedures. Thus, surgical therapy of benign brain tumors and its advantages and disadvantages should be thoroughly discussed with patients and their relatives to ensure that the therapeutic concept represents ethical decision-making with core benefits to the patients.

Spinal Disorders in Very Old Patients

As life expectancy is increasing along with accelerating improvements in patients' QoL and the health-care system, it is expected that the proportion of the world's population over the age of sixty will nearly double, from 12 percent to 22 percent from 2015 to 2025.[25] Aging can substantially affect all spinal elements, including the intervertebral discs, facet joints, and supporting muscles and ligaments, leading to biomechanical alterations and anatomical changes. Such degenerative changes might result in spinal and foraminal narrowing, thereby significantly compressing the vascular and neural structures of the spinal cord, reflected clinically as neurogenic claudication or lumbar radiculopathy. These conditions could cause a decrease in the mobility and QoL of elderly patients.

There is no clear consensus on the optimal treatment for octogenarians (patients in their eighties), especially in cases of instability. This raises the question whether older frail patients should be treated conservatively. My colleagues and I (Unterberg) found that neurological improvement and mortality rates after simple decompression and the more complex fusion surgeries were similar and relatively low, even in patients aged eighty and older.[26] Similar findings were also reported in octogenarians with spinal infections.[27] Spinal infection is a dev-

---

[24] Stepan Fedorko, Klaus Zweckberger, and Andreas W. Unterberg, "Quality of Life Following Surgical Treatment of Lesions within the Pineal Region," *Journal of Neurosurgery* 130 (2018): 28–37, https://doi.org/10.3171/2017.7.JNS17260.

[25] Fehlings et al., "The Aging of the Global Population."

[26] Pavlina Lenga et al., "Lumbar Decompression versus Decompression and Fusion in Octogenarians: Complications and Clinical Course With 3-Year Follow-Up," *Global Spine Journal*, Sep. 23, 2022, https://doi.org/10.1177/21925682221121099.

[27] Pavlina Lenga et al., "Decompression only versus Fusion in Octogenarians with Spinal Epidural Abscesses: Early Complications, Clinical and Radiological Outcome with 2-

astating disease associated with high morbidity and mortality rates, especially in older patients. As my colleagues and I showed in our case series on octogenarians with a spinal infection, even such a cohort with frailty could benefit from surgery, with a significant amelioration of their functional status and mitigation of related mortality rates.[28] The same study group also compared octogenarians with younger patients from sixty-five to seventy-nine years of age and concluded that surgery led to better outcomes in all age groups.[29] Even in the case of spinal tumors, such as meningiomas, surgery seems to be the preferred approach, even in this debilitating cohort.[30] Thus, even in very old and frail patients, emergency and elective spinal surgery is of considerable benefit.

Perspectives and Conclusions

Surgical ethics is an essential component of surgical practice. Even the most technically skilled surgeons who perform successful surgeries require an ethical approach. The role of a surgeon is also paramount to ensure quality management of patients. Surgeons should be skilled in surgery but also ethically trustworthy. They must recognize that the nature of surgical work provides fertile ground in which ethical problems can grow, and thus they need to be aware of and prepared for ethical issues. Surgeons should rely upon their judgment and their values and beliefs to make ethical decisions and, if necessary, to take difficult decisions to an ethical consultation or committee. An interdisciplinary approach is sometimes mandatory to provide the most beneficial and safest therapy for patients with complex pathologies, such as brain or spinal tumors. Thus, education at the trainee level is important not only for learning an ethical approach to medical problems but also for learning to work harmoniously with colleagues from other disciplines, with the main goal being beneficence for patients and not financial or scientific gains. A "good surgeon" should be defined by professional responsibilities or values, such as empathy, honesty, integrity, dedication, devotion, nondiscrimination, compassion, ethics, and professionalism, which form a physician's identity.

Year Follow-Up," *Neurosurgery Review* (2022), https://doi.org/10.1007/s10143-022-01805-4.

[28] Ibid.

[29] Pavlina Lenga et al., "Lumbar Decompression versus Decompression and Fusion in Octogenarians."

[30] Pavlina Lenga et al., "Spinal Meningioma Surgery in Octogenarians: Functional Outcomes and Complications over a 2-Year Follow-Up Period," *Medicina* (Kaunas, Lithuania) 58 (2022): 1481, https://doi.org/10.3390/medicina58101481.

Furthermore, the balance between technical skills and ethical reasoning makes a good surgeon. Ethics education can contribute to making surgeons more competent. It can also make them better prepared to make ethical decisions on issues encountered in daily practice, in the application of new technologies, and in a surgical environment that is increasingly institutionalized and under economic pressure. Community and institutional standards can be created proactively to establish evaluation criteria that define or recognize futile surgeries and a process for addressing futility claims case by case. The value of surgery can be evaluated based on the outcomes and benefits delivered by the procedure. A mere economic evaluation is inappropriate when discussing the value of surgery. Quality is more difficult to assess than value. Structural, process, and outcome measures should be used as quality indicators. It is important to implement a composite scoring system during surgery. The procedure itself might be the most important factor when determining the most effective approach for quality assessment. Other quality assessment measures, including complications, especially surgical site infections, mortality, postsurgical QoL scores, should be used as well. Adequately powered, high-quality studies, from descriptive to diagnostic to interventional, are needed to improve the quality and length of patients' lives. High-risk surgeries are a part of the daily routine; therefore, sufficient preoperative preparation of both surgeons and patients is essential to achieve the best outcomes. While postoperative complication rates are high, modern technologies should be employed to preserve patients' functionality rather than for the neurosurgeons' own scientific or financial gains.

Decision-making can be very difficult; however, it should be guided by respect for the patient's autonomy, informed consent, beneficence, nonmaleficence, and justice. Surgery should not be conceived merely as an applied technological practice but as an ethical healing art!

In conclusion, ethics should be present and promoted in all neurosurgical sectors. Financial profits or personal ambitions associated with the industrialization processes taking place in medicine should be absent. Professionalism as well as ethics in decision-making are an essential part of the daily neurosurgical life and represent traits that should be established already from day one in residents' training.

Part Three:
Digital Medicine and Ethical Decisions

Ethical Aspects of Digital Transformation in Medicine and Health Care

Giovanni Rubeis and Nadia Primc

1. Introduction

Digitalization of medicine and health care is a topic of growing public interest that covers a large range of applications and affects all areas of health care. Digital health tools include electronic health records, mobile health apps and digital platforms (mHealth), telemedicine, the use of sensors and wearables to track physiological parameters and the general well-being of users, robots, and the use of artificial intelligence (AI) and big data in diagnostics, treatment decision, and scientific research. Digitalization is discussed as a promising strategy in dealing with current and future challenges in health care, namely, demographic change and growing health-care needs, rising costs, and the increasing shortage of health-care professionals. Great hopes and fears are associated with digitalization, the fears mainly relating to potential negative impact on fundamental ethical values in health care.

A recurrent misunderstanding in the public debate is that every form of digitization represents a form of digital transformation—for example, that the implementation of digital technologies automatically implies a digital transformation of health care. This expectation is often based on the characterization of digital technologies, especially AI, as disruptive, without questioning what exactly the disruptive or transformative nature of digital technologies is. Digital transformation has become "a hype and buzzword in both academic and practitioner literatures."[1] Furthermore, the terms digital transformation, digitalization, and digitization are sometimes used interchangeably. Digital transformation has become an "umbrella-concept coined in order to cover automation, mechanization, ma-

---

[1] Chen Gong and Vincent Ribiere, "Developing a Unified Definition of Digital Transformation," *Technovation* 102, no. 102217 (Apr. 2021): 1, https://doi.org/10.1016/j.technovation.2020.102217.

chinization, robotization" as well as data-driven technologies.[2] However, digital transformation does not simply take place by replacing analog technologies with digital ones—for example, replacing telefax or paper-based medical charts with digital communication and documentation tools (email, electronic health records)—as long as the underlying health-care processes remain the same. The confusion in the use of the term is further promoted by the fact that different academic disciplines and stakeholders (IT, health economics, administration, health-care disciplines, ethics) have different perspectives and interests in the digital transformation of the health-care sector.

In this chapter, we first give a more detailed account of the term "digital transformation," arguing that it is to be understood as a normative concept, which from an ethical point of view is to be measured by the extent to which digital technologies can actually contribute to improved health care. In doing so, we use the four principles of Tom Beauchamp and James Childress as an overarching normative framework.[3] In a further step, we take a closer look at these ethical principles regarding different digital technologies currently applied or developed in the field of medicine and health care. Finally, we discuss strategies for enabling successful digital transformation of healthcare guided by fundamental ethical values and principles.

2. Digitization, Digitalization, Digital Transformation, and the Digital Disruption of Health Care

Digitization, digitalization, digital transformation, and the disruptive nature of digital technologies are closely interrelated terms focussing on different aspects of the increasing use of digital health technologies. We use "digitization" to denote the technological process of converting information from an analog to a digital form. "Digitalization" goes beyond the technological process of digitization and encompasses using digital technologies to optimize processes and generate better outcomes.[4] Digitalization, hence, designates a sociotechnological process, as the implementation of digital technologies usually implies changes in organizational or societal structures (for example, changes in access to health data, or in the doctor-patient relationship) as well as process outcomes (for example, better diagnostics and more personalized treatment), or even generation of new

---

[2] Peter G. Kirchenschlaeger, *Digital Transformation and Ethics: Ethical Considerations on the Robotization and Automation of Society and the Economy and the Use of Artificial Intelligence* (Baden-Baden: Nomos, 2021), 107–08.

[3] Tom L. Beauchamp and James F. Childress, *Principles of Biomedical Ethics* (New York: Oxford University Press, 2019).

[4] Gong and Ribiere, "Developing a Unified Definition of Digital Transformation," 9.

health-care products and services (for example, mHealth applications and telemedicine). This also includes the expectation that digitization will contribute to an overall improvement of processes and/or outcomes.

While digitization and digitalization can be differentiated relatively well, the distinction between digitalization and "digital transformation" is more difficult. Digital transformation emphasizes the aspect of change, which is already part of the concept of digitalization. Hence, while "all transformation is change, not all change is transformation. Transformation needs to meet the criteria of the three 'Bs'—it must be Big, must be Bold (i.e., the intensity and degree of change involved), and lead to Better outcomes."[5] Digitalization of health care thus signifies the process of incremental change and (intended) improvement of health care by implementing digital technologies that may lead to digital transformation, that is, a fundamental change and radical improvement of the quality of health care. We will address the aspects of fundamental change and improvement of quality separately.

Since digital transformation describes a change that is deemed radical, this partly explains why digital transformation is often linked to the characterization of digital technologies as disruptive. However, the disruptive nature of technologies or innovations is often not defined appropriately, which leads to a circular reasoning, insofar as the disruptive nature of digital technologies is defined as their potential to bring about a digital transformation, and the digital transformation in turn is the result of the disruptive nature of digitalization. The concept of disruptive innovation originates in business theory and was introduced by Joseph Bower and Clayton Christensen.[6] The concept was initially designed to explain why some incumbent and leading companies fail to adapt to innovations initially offered by new or small companies to the low-end customers of an established market or to customers of a new market, and which in the further development then push the established companies out of their own business field. Different strategies are discussed as to how established providers can react to potentially disruptive innovations in order to secure their own success and market position. One possibility (which will be relevant for our further investigation) is for the leading companies to become developers of potentially disruptive innovations themselves, or to integrate potentially disruptive innovations into their own business strategy at an early stage.[7]

As the idea of disruptive innovations was originally developed in the field of business theory with the aim to serve very specific epistemological and practical

---

[5] Ibid.

[6] Joseph L. Bower and Clayton M. Christensen, "Disruptive Technologies: Catching the Wave," *Harvard Business Review* 73, no. 1 (Jan.-Feb. 1995): 43–53.

[7] Clayton M. Christensen, Michael Raynor, and Rory McDonald, "What Is Disruptive Innovation?," *Harvard Business Review* 93, no. 12 (Dec. 2015): 44–53.

goals, it cannot be easily transferred to the field of medicine and health care. We still believe that general conclusions can be drawn for ethical discussion. First, digitalization can be seen as potentially disruptive, especially if it is developed by stakeholders (domain experts) outside the health-care sector specifically aiming for increasing efficiency and reducing costs. This gradually forces health-care professionals and patients to adapt to the requirements of these technological developments instead of technological developments adapting to the needs and values of professionals and patients. This process is sometimes referred to as technology push. From an ethical point of view, the digitalization of health care is disruptive when well-grounded, fundamental values and ethical principles of health care are increasingly pushed into the background by technological developments, or are (at least partly) replaced by new ones. Second, the potentially disruptive nature of digitalization can be counteracted by including the needs of health-care professionals and patients in the technological development. Such participatory approaches are needed to ensure that digitalization leads to a change that actually means a significant improvement of quality of health care—which leads us to the second aspect of the definition of digital transformation.

If digital transformation designates not so much any radical change but primarily a qualitative improvement of health care, then the question arises as to which criteria should be used to determine and measure quality of health care. On one hand, such criteria include the empirical evaluation of the digital applications using relevant clinical endpoints, surrogate parameters, and further health-care-related quality indicators. On the other hand, they also require a normative and ethical assessment, that is, the question to what extent digital applications consider, strengthen, or weaken certain values and ethical aspects of medicine and health care.

Given the variety of ethical approaches in the field of biomedical ethics, we use the approach of Tom Beauchamp and James Childress as a normative framework to discuss essential ethical aspects of digitalized health care.[8] Beauchamp and Childress identify four clusters of principles that are generally accepted as fundamental norms in biomedical ethics, namely, respect for autonomy, nonmaleficence, beneficence, and justice. Although Beauchamp and Childress insist that the principles of nonmaleficence and beneficence should be analyzed separately and not conflated into a single principle,[9] we will (for reasons of brevity) discuss the two principles together in our consideration of the potential benefits and risks of digitalized health care for the well-being of patients. Hence, we ar-

---

[8] Beauchamp and Childress, *Principles of Biomedical Ethics*.
[9] They rightly point out that the obligation to not harm (nonmaleficence) is not the same as the obligation to help (beneficence); see Beauchamp and Childress, *Principles of Biomedical Ethics*, 156.

gue that, from an ethical point of view, digital transformation should be understood as a normative concept that designates the quest to significantly strengthen the autonomy of patients, enhance the well-being of patients, and minimize inequalities in access to health care and health status through the implementation of digital tools. Digital transformation is to be understood as a continuous challenge to achieve and ensure these goals, and not just as a result of digitalization. Disruption, on the other hand, takes place when these goals and fundamental values of medicine and health care are put at risk by the process of digitalization.

3. Autonomy as a Goal and Prerequisite for Digitalization of Medicine and Health Care

Autonomy plays a crucial role in the debate on digital health technologies. First, it can be seen as a prerequisite for the use of these technologies, that is, the capability of self-determined decision-making and action. Second, the purpose of digital technologies may be to empower users and to (re)establish their autonomy. Since we cannot discuss this very complex matter in regard to all digital health technologies, we will focus on two fields of application that illustrate the potentials and challenges of these technologies in the context of autonomy. Our examples are mobile health (mHealth) technologies and assistive technologies that include monitoring systems and sensors. On one hand, these technologies are meant not only to improve the quality of health-care services but also to empower patients through their use. On the other hand, a certain degree of autonomy, that is, being able to decide and act independently, is needed in order to be able to use these technologies.

3.1 Autonomy as Participation: The Example of mHealth

Mobile health (mHealth) technologies are often believed to have the potential to transform the power dynamic between patients and doctors. According to some authors, mHealth empowers patients because it gives them the opportunity to actively participate in the treatment process.[10] By using smart wearable sensors as well as health apps for smartphones and tablets, patients may track their in-

---

[10] Eric Topol, *The Creative Destruction of Medicine: How the Digital Revolution Will Create Better Health Care* (New York: Basic Books, 2013); Eric Topol, *The Patient Will See You Now: The Future of Medicine Is in Your Hands* (New York: Basic Books, 2015); Eric Topol, *Deep Medicine: How Artificial Intelligence Can Make Healthcare Human Again* (New York: Basic Books, 2019).

dividual health data from vital functions to behavioral patterns (eating habits, exercise, sleep). The data generated by patients can be either transmitted passively via telemetry to health professionals or actively documented and communicated to health professionals by the patients themselves. Thus, patients may gain knowledge about their health and take control over their own health data. Some authors consider this as empowerment, since the active participation of better-informed patients implies a shift in the power relation between patients and health professionals.[11] Patients are no longer passive recipients of information and therapeutic advice, but play an active role in collecting relevant data and making health-related decisions.

More critical voices state that this view is oversimplified, since it ignores the fact that whether mHealth is considered as an empowerment largely depends on the concept of autonomy one refers to.[12] A crucial differentiation in this regard is the distinction between the autonomy of consumers and that of patients. Consumers use mHealth applications without a medical indication, that is, for lifestyle purposes like losing weight or strengthening their well-being. In this context, autonomy might just mean taking health matters into one's own hands and gaining control over certain health data. Patients, however, might be in a vulnerable position, thus needing more sophisticated forms of guidance and support when using these applications. They also need more in-depth patient information and contact with health professionals during the use of mHealth technologies. Thus, the requirements and preconditions of enacting one's autonomy, mainly a solid information basis, may differ between consumers and patients. When patients use apps that are not suited for them or use them without the proper information, this might undermine their autonomy instead of empowering it.[13]

Other commentators question the framing of empowerment in the context of mHealth altogether. Jessica Morley and Luciano Floridi[14] state that identifying mHealth with empowerment rests on claims that lack empirical evidence. According to their approach, two aspects contradict the empowerment view. First, the two aspects of autonomy—as a goal and as a prerequisite—turn out to be problematic and may actually conflict with each other. Furthermore, individual needs, requirements, and context may vary drastically between users. Given this

---

[11] Topol, *The Patient Will See You Now*.

[12] Bettina Schmietow and Georg Marckmann, "Mobile Health Ethics and the Expanding Role of Autonomy," *Medicine, Health Care and Philosophy* 22, no. 4 (Dec. 2019): 623–30, https://doi.org/10.1007/s11019-019-09900-y.

[13] Ibid.

[14] Jessica Morley and Luciano Floridi, "The Limits of Empowerment: How to Reframe the Role of mHealth Tools in the Healthcare Ecosystem," *Science and Engineering Ethics* 26, no. 3 (Jun. 2020): 1159–83, https://doi.org/10.1007/s11948-019-00115-1.

complexity, one cannot simply claim that the use of mHealth means an empowerment in every case. In addition, the level of health literacy, that is, the ability to understand health-related information, also varies between users. That means that not all users are capable of processing health-related data and making autonomous decisions based on them in the same way. Therefore, Morley and Floridi suggest understanding mHealth applications as "digital companions," meaning instruments for supporting patients instead of tools of empowerment.

In addition to not fulfilling the supposed purpose of empowerment, mHealth technologies may pose an actual danger to autonomy. One of the most important aspects in this regard is the potential of self-tracking and self-monitoring as tools of disciplining.[15] The use of mHealth is most efficient when patients track and monitor as many individual health data as possible, ideally in their daily living. This means that medical technology dissolves the borders between the medical realm and the private sphere. The ubiquitous and permanent surveillance may be used not only to generate data but also to actively direct the behavior of patients. For example, an app for documenting dietary habits and exercise to predict and prevent cardiovascular disease may be used not primarily for the patient's benefit, but for enforcing a behavior that primarily contributes to reducing public health costs. As a result, patients adapt to routines dictated by technology for reasons that might not be in their interest. Such an app could be used for implementing a certain health agenda and thus may be a tool for further advancing the desolidarization process within the health sector by shifting responsibilities toward the individual. Thus, health increasingly becomes an individual responsibility. In this regard, autonomy and empowerment are simply rhetorical devices to obscure a hidden agenda.

Furthermore, it is unclear whether mHealth may lead to a shift in power relations in the doctor-patient relationship. While some see the potential for democratizing this relationship,[16] others state that the overreliance on quantifiable

---

[15] Btihaj Ajana, "Digital Health and the Biopolitics of the Quantified Self," *Digital Health* 3 (Feb. 2017), https://doi.org/10.1177/2055207616689509; Deborah Lupton, "Self-Tracking, Health and Medicine," *Health Sociology Review* 26, no. 1 (2017): 1–5; Deborah Lupton, *The Quantified Self. A Sociology of Self-Tracking* (Cambridge: Polity Press, 2016); Deborah Lupton, "The Digitally Engaged Patient: Self-Monitoring and Self-Care in the Digital Health Era," *Social Theory & Health* 11, no. 3 (Jun. 2013): 256–70.

[16] Topol, *The Creative Destruction of Medicine*; Topol, *Deep Medicine*; Bonyan Qudaha and Karen Luetsch, "The Influence of Mobile Health Applications on Patient-Healthcare Provider Relationships: A Systematic, Narrative Review," *Patient Education and Counseling* 102, no. 6 (Jun. 2019), 1080–89, https://doi.org/10.1016/j.pec.2019.01.021.

data may lead to a dehumanization of the clinical encounter.[17] It is also highly questionable whether implementing technology alone may democratize relations without changing the framework of the social practices in question.[18] This is especially the case since regulatory issues concerning patient and data security are often unclear. Thus, expectations of a power shift and democratization are exaggerated, since they focus only on the technology and ignore the social and relational aspects of its use.[19]

3.2 Supporting Autonomy: Assistive Technologies

Assistive technologies offer a wide range of applications, from assisting older adults in their daily activities to supporting rehabilitation. These technologies encompass monitoring and surveillance systems, smart sensors, and robotics. One of the major fields of application is ambient assisted living (AAL), where smart home systems (sensors, monitoring, internet of things) are combined with surveillance systems and ubiquitous computing, sometimes also robotics.[20] AAL aims at enabling older adults or people with special needs to live as independently as possible in their own home.[21] For example, these systems may monitor heating, gas, and water consumption for security purposes, detect abnormal gait pattern through smart floor sensors and thus detect falls, or recognize and regulate the emotions of users by using facial recognition. Besides enabling an in-

---

[17] Carlo Botrugno, "Information Technologies in Healthcare: Enhancing or Dehumanising Doctor–Patient Interaction?," *Health* 25, no. 4 (Jul. 2021): 475–93, https://doi.org/10.1177/1363459319891213.

[18] Anita Ho and Oliver Quick, "Leaving Patients to Their Own Devices? Smart Technology, Safety and Therapeutic Relationships," *BMC Medical Ethics* 19, no. 1 (Mar. 2018): 18, https://doi.org/0.1186/s12910-018-0255-8.

[19] Giovanni Rubeis, Keerthi Dubbala Keerthi, and Ingrid Metzle, "'Democratizing' Artificial Intelligence in Medicine and Healthcare: Mapping the Uses of an Elusive Term," *Frontiers in Genetics* 15, no. 13 (Aug. 2022): 902542, https://doi.org/10.3389/fgene.2022.902542.

[20] A. Hasan Sapci and H. Aylin Sapci, "Innovative Assisted Living Tools, Remote Monitoring Technologies, Artificial Intelligence-Driven Solutions, and Robotic Systems for Aging Societies: Systematic Review," *JMIR Aging* 2, no. 2 (Nov. 2019): e15429, https://doi.org/10.2196/15429; Andrew Sixsmith, "Technology and the Challenge of Aging," in *Technologies for Active Aging: International Perspectives on Aging*, ed. Andrew Sixsmith and Gloria Gutman (Boston: Springer, 2013), 7–25.

[21] Craig Kuziemsky et al., "Role of Artificial Intelligence within the Telehealth Domain," *Yearbook of Medical Informatics* 28, no. 1 (Apr. 2019): 35–40, https://doi.org/10.1055/s-0039-1677897.

tersectoral cooperation and data exchange and ensuring safety at home, the explicit aim of AAL is to preserve or improve the quality of life of users.[22]

Autonomy, understood as being able to perform activities of daily living mostly interdependently, is mostly a goal in assistive technologies, not so much a prerequisite. Users do not interact with many of these applications systems, since they are running more in the background. This unobtrusiveness is in fact a crucial feature of many assistive technologies. This very fact may become a problem for autonomy. Users may not be aware that they are interacting with automated systems and nonhuman agents. Smart systems may function automatically and not respond to users' requests, which may undermine autonomous decision-making and action.

Again, the concept of autonomy behind these technologies is crucial. As we have seen, autonomy is mostly framed as being able to live an independent life in one's own home. Although independent living may be seen as one aspect of autonomy, it is not the only or even the crucial goal. The ability and possibility to make self-determined, well-informed decisions is far more important than whether an individual lives is their own apartment. But the issues go further —the very technologies that enable independent living at home might undermine autonomy in a fuller sense. Monitoring and sensor technologies imply an intrusion into privacy and permanent surveillance.[23] This intrusion does not mean the violation of some abstract notion of privacy, but it can have concrete effects. The feeling of being permanently watched may enforce a certain behavior by the users. This form of disciplining[24] may be an unwanted result of surveillance. It may also be a strategy for enforcing conformity and nudging people into a certain behavior that might not correspond with their own choices and needs. This is especially the case since users seldom have a say in the design and implementation of these technologies. Leading an active, independent life alone in an apartment is a choice that has already been made for them. Whether being cared for by machines is what these people want is also not a matter of their choosing. Reducing autonomy to independent living therefore evokes a conflict between

---

[22] Alexandra Queirós et al., "Ambient Assisted Living and Health-Related Outcomes—A Systematic Literature Review," *Informatics* 4, no. 3 (Jul. 2017): 19, https://doi.org/10.3390/informatics4030019.

[23] Nabile M. Safdar, John D. Banja, and Carolyn C. Meltzer, "Ethical Considerations in Artificial Intelligence," *European Journal of Radiology* 122 (Jan. 2020): 108768, https://doi.org/ 10.1016/j.ejrad.2019.108768.

[24] W. Ben Mortenson, Andrew Sixsmith, and Ryan Woolrych, "The Power(s) of Observation: Theoretical Perspectives on Surveillance Technologies and Older People," *Ageing & Society* 35, no. 3 (Mar. 2015): 512–35, https://doi.org/10.1017/S0144686X13000 846.

the intended empowerment and the disempowering effects these technologies may have.

Assistive technologies and mHealth illustrate the disruptive potential of digitalized healthcare when it comes to autonomy. There is a risk that these technologies require or aim for types of autonomy that are either oversimplified or misguided. These technologies may therefore either fail to empower the autonomy of patients or even undermine it by substituting something that is similar, but not quite the same: self-tracking as a form of controlling one's own health in the case of mHealth, or independent living at home in the case of assistive technologies.

4. Benefits and Risks of Digitalization for the Well-Being of Patients

One of the areas where digital technologies have shown promising results is diagnostics and decision support. Machine learning and data mining are used to detect patterns in large data sets, extracting relevant information and combining it with data from other sources.[25] It is thus possible to find significant associations within the data—for example, the correlation between a cancer diagnosis and survival. It is also possible to evaluate the quality of data and measure their predictive power. These approaches allow a more precise diagnostics as well as better ways of predictive data analytics, which is especially relevant for disease prevention and early interventions. Disease progression can be modeled, and the risk of disease onset can be predicted more precisely. But the possibilities of these system go beyond improving diagnostics and prognosis. In clinical decision support systems (CDSS), these technologies may assist health professionals in making sense of diagnostic data and finding the best treatment option.[26] Google's Deep Mind was capable of outperforming human practitioners in detecting breast cancer in mammography and reducing the workload for practitioners by up to 88 percent.[27] IBM's Watson for Oncology was fed with thousands of real cancer cases and given the task of suggesting a treatment option. A meta-anal-

---

[25] Giovanni Briganti and Olivier Le Moine, "Artificial Intelligence in Medicine: Today and Tomorrow," *Frontiers in Medicine* 7, no. 27 (Feb. 2020): https://doi.org/10.3389/fmed.2020.00027.

[26] F. Amisha et al., "Overview of Artificial Intelligence in Medicine," *Journal of Family Medicine and Primary Care* 8, no. 7 (Jul. 2019): 2328–31, https://doi.org/10.4103/jfpmc.jfmpc_440_19.

[27] Scott Mayer McKinney et al., "International Evaluation of an AI System for Breast Cancer Screening," *Nature* 577 (Jan. 2020): 89–94, https://doi.org/10.1038/s41586-019-1799-6.

ysis of published studies comes to the conclusion that the system's suggestions to treat or to more closely consider patients for cancer treatments matched with the suggestions of multidisciplinary teams on average in 81.52 percent of cases, although the concordance rate seems to vary for different types and stages of cancer.[28] The difference is that Watson can come up with a suggestion in a matter of minutes by integrating data from the case with all available scientific data, something no human could do. Patients could thus benefit immensely from digitally enhanced diagnostics and CDSS due to the precision, speed, and efficiency of these systems.

The introduction of nonhuman actors into the clinical encounter raises a variety of ethical issues. First, the ontological and moral status of these actors is unclear. If we consider them as moral agents, it would have far-reaching implications in an ethical as well as legal sense.[29] Can computer systems be morally or legally responsible for mistakes? Can they be held accountable for malpractice? Second, deprofessionalization might occur, since these systems may negatively affect the autonomy and agency of health professionals, which may also affect the doctor-patient-relationship.[30] Third, the so-called black box phenomenon—that is, the opacity of machine learning processes—may also complicate the information process, since health professionals may not always be able to fully explain how a decision was made by a computer. As a result, it may be more difficult for patients to trust in digitally enhanced decisions, which is especially relevant since trust is a fundamental element in the doctor-patient relationship.

In conclusion, smart diagnostic systems and CDSS may be crucial tools for improving the well-being of patients. Due to their ability to combine, process, and analyze large amounts of data from different sources, as well as their precision and speed, these technologies enable a more personalized treatment. However, there is also the potential for disrupting clinical practices and relations. The expertise of health-care professionals and personal relations are cornerstones of trust within the clinical encounter. Introducing a new actor without a clearly defined set of responsibilities whose decisions and actions cannot be fully explained can hamper the willingness of patients to trust health profession-

---

[28] Zhou Jie, Zeng Zhiying, and Li Li, "A Meta-Analysis of Watson for Oncology in Clinical Application," *Scientific Reports* 11, no. 5792 (Mar. 2021): https://doi.org/10.1038/s41598-021-84973-5.

[29] Sally Dalton-Brown, "The Ethics of Medical AI and the Physician-Patient Relationship," *Cambridge Quarterly of Healthcare Ethics* 29, no. 1 (Jan. 2020): 115–21, https://doi.org/10.1017/S0963180119000847.

[30] Mark Henderson Arnold, "Teasing out Artificial Intelligence in Medicine: An Ethical Critique of Artificial Intelligence and Machine Learning in Medicine," *Bioethical Inquiry* 18 (Jan. 2019): 121–39, https://doi.org/10.1007/s11673-020-10080-1.

als. This may lead to a dehumanized health care in which patients are increasingly confronted with automated processes and faceless actors.

5. Issues of Justice and Inequalities in Digitalized Health Care

One of the crucial benefits of digital health technologies is the ability to integrate huge amounts of data from different sources. A person's genetic information, environmental situation, and behavioral information can be combined in order to get a fuller, more detailed picture of their health. This allows a more personalized treatment as well as a better prediction of health risks. This big-data approach to health implies quantification and datafication of all relevant areas of a person's life. In order to do that, two processes are crucial: datafication, which means transforming all relevant information into a quantifiable, standardized format that can be processed by smart computers; and defining biomarkers, that is, indicators that allow measuring, predicting, or evaluating health-related outcomes.[31] Thus, the main task of personalization is to find traits that may serve as viable indicators for health and illness and quantify the information based on them so that it can be used for standardized analysis.

A fundamental risk of the big-data approach is the epistemic overestimation or misconception of what data are. Digital positivism[32] refers to the view that data speak for themselves and possess an inherent meaning that just needs to be analyzed. The epistemological superiority of quantified and standardized data over human observation and judgment is also seen as an opportunity to get rid of bias and make health care more equitable. However, digital positivism ignores the fact that data are socially constructed and embedded. The power relations and agency of key stakeholders as well as the social context from which data are taken is therefore crucial for assessing their value, validity, and true scope. In order to make sense of data, one has to consider the social practices of data collection and utilization against the backdrop of corporate, institutional, and governmental structures.[33]

From this point of view, the selection of biomarkers as well as the standardization of data might become problematic, since it may ignore the specific needs

---

[31] Nicole L Guthrie et al., "Emergence of Digital Biomarkers to Predict and Modify Treatment Efficacy: Machine Learning Study," *BMJ Open* 9, no. 7 (Jul. 2019), e030710, http://dx.doi.org/10.1136/bmjopen-2019-030710.

[32] Vincent Mosco, *To the Cloud: Big Data in a Turbulent World* (Boulder, Colo.: Paradigm, 2015).

[33] Annika Richterich, *The Big Data Agenda: Data Ethics and Critical Data Studies* (London: University of Westminster Press, 2018).

and resources of certain groups and individuals. One reason is that the need for clear-cut biomarkers poses the risk of decontextualizing these parameters from their social determinants. In health care, we see that certain traits associated with ethnicity or gender are taken as biological facts. This is true in some regards. For example, symptoms of cardiac arrest vary between the sexes. Women show other symptoms than men, but since the male anatomy and physiology are still the standard in medicine, women's symptoms are often overlooked. On the other hand, some traits associated with a certain group are not inherently linked to ethnicity or gender. Instead, these traits exist as a result of structural racism or sexism. One striking example is hypertension in black people.[34] The prevalence of hypertension and health conditions associated with it, such as diabetes or kidney failure, is significantly higher in black people than in the rest of the population. The reason is not genetic; rather, systematic discrimination manifest in poor housing, low socioeconomic standard, denial of access to health care and education, and the mental stressors linked to these factors contribute to a lifestyle that causes hypertension.[35]

Regarding justice, this means that a big-data approach may contribute to a more personalized health care, thus improving access and health equity. However, the focus on big amounts of data alone does not guarantee the inclusion of marginalized groups and the elimination of bias. It may even undermine the very goal of justice when the context and social determinants shaping data and the practices of data collection and utilization are ignored. Thus, the increasing focus on quantifiable and standardized data might be disruptive, since it perpetuates or aggravates health inequalities as well bias.

6. Strategies to Promote Digital Transformation and Prevent a Digital Disruption in Medicine and Health Care

As we have seen, despite their great potential for improving health-care practices and benefitting patients, digital health technologies may negatively affect established values, that is, have a disruptive impact on health care. Challenges arise mainly because the technologies in question are often based on oversim-

---

[34] Nwamaka D. Eneanya, Sophia Kostelanetz, and Mallika L Mendu, "Race-Free Biomarkers to Quantify Kidney Function: Health Equity Lessons Learned from Population-Based Research," *American Journal of Kidney Diseases* 77, no. 5 (May 2021): 667–69, https://doi.org/10.1053/j.ajkd.2020.12.001.

[35] Alicia Lukachko, Mark L. Hatzenbuehler, and Katherine M. Keyes, "Structural Racism and Myocardial Infarction in the United States," *Social Science & Medicine* 103 (Feb. 2014): 42–50, https://doi.org/10.1016/j.socscimed.2013.07.021.

plified assumptions and ignore the complexity of social practices and relations in the health-care setting. In order to address these challenges, we suggest several strategies that aim for a more nuanced, context-sensitive design, implementation, and use of digital health technologies.

6.1 Participatory Technology Design

Models of participatory design of health technology strive for including all relevant stakeholders in the development process.[36] This implies integrating the perspective of patients and users, health professionals, and other possible actors (relatives, policy makers, health-insurance agencies). The aim is to ensure that a technology fits with the needs and resources of those who interact with it, use it, or are otherwise affected by it. One advantage of this approach is that it enables technology designers to integrate different types knowledge, such as medical as well as nursing expertise and first-person accounts of patients. Since designers often do not have domain expertise, participatory design can bridge this knowledge gap. It also allows inclusion of knowledge that goes beyond fact-based domain knowledge, that is, the intricacies of social practices and relations. Besides ensuring that health technologies fulfill the promise of personalization, this approach may also empower patients by giving them the opportunity to actively participate in the design process.

6.2 Diversifying Data

As we have seen, decontextualized data that are detached from their social determinants may create a severe risk. One way to deal with this risk is to assess and evaluate the data based on the degree of the context sensitivity and inclusiveness they represent. This means actively preferring data sets—for example, as training data for algorithms—that make social determinants explicit.[37] In addition, it is crucial to make the underlying parameters of an algorithm-based sys-

---

[36] Pieter Vandekerckhove et al., "Generative Participatory Design Methodology to Develop Electronic Health Interventions: Systematic Literature Review," *Journal of Medical Internet Research* 22, no. 4 (Apr. 2020): e13780, https://doi.org/10.2196/13780.

[37] Colin G. Walsh et al., "Stigma, Biomarkers, and Algorithmic Bias: Recommendations for Precision Behavioral Health with Artificial Intelligence," *JAMIA Open* 3, no. 1 (Jan. 2020): 9–15, https://doi.org/10.1093/jamiaopen/ooz054.

tem transparent.[38] This implies explaining why certain parameters—for example, biomarkers—are deemed relevant and thus disclose the interpretative framework used for a certain application.

6.3 Improving eHealth Literacy

Literacy in eHealth refers to the ability to deal with digital health information and applications. Several models for training these abilities have been suggested and proven to be successful—for example, trainer-focused approaches or shared learning.[39] These models focus on two crucial aspects: skills for handling digital health technologies, and the ability to assess and evaluate health-related information. An improved eHealth literacy may contribute to a better acceptance of digital health technologies and thus contribute to realizing their full potential.

7. Conclusion

We have argued that digital transformation of medicine and health care should be understood as a normative term that designates a fundamental change and radical improvement of quality of health care through the process of digitalization. Any attempt to significantly improve the overall quality of health-care needs to consider the fundamental ethical values in the field of medicine and health care, namely, the respect of the autonomy of patients, the promotion of well-being of patients, as well as the prevention of inequalities between patients. Digital transformation can be achieved only by integrating these values in the process of digitalization. We have presented some strategies that can help to promote such an ethically reflected process of digitalization.

Given the big impact that digitalization is supposed to have on the fields of medicine and health care, it has been proposed to revise the Hippocratic Oath for the era of digitalized health care. This revision would acknowledge the technology-related changes in the future and culture of health care and help prevent a digital disruption of health care primarily associated with the fears of a growing deprofessionalization and dehumanization of health care: "I will remember that

---

[38] Milena A. Gianfrancesco et al., "Potential Biases in Machine Learning Algorithms Using Electronic Health Record Data," *JAMA International Medicine* 178, no. 11 (Nov. 2018), 1544–47, https://doi.org/10.1001/jamainternmed.2018.3763.

[39] Sara Pourrazavi et al., "Theory-Based E-health Literacy Interventions in Older Adults: A Systematic Review," *Archives of Public Health* 78, no. 72 (Aug. 2020), https://doi.org/10.1186/s13690-020-00455-6.

I do not treat a fever chart, a cancerous growth, a data point, or an algorithm's suggestion, but a human being."[40]

---

[40] Bertalan Mesko and Brennan Spiegel, "A Revised Hippocratic Oath for the Era of Digital Health," *Journal of Medical Internet Research* 24, no. 9 (Sep. 2022): e39177, https://doi.org/10.2196/39177.

Family Decision-Making in Times of Genomic Newborn Screening

Beate Ditzen and Christian P. Schaaf

Introduction

For an increasing number of diseases and disease predispositions, genetic causes have been identified. This provides individuals and families with the possibility of learning more about hereditary predictors and genetic susceptibility for known disorders or clinical manifestations, which would otherwise remain undetermined. This has been implemented in clinical practice through genetic testing of affected individuals, and subsequent predictive or presymptomatic testing of their family members. Since more recently, genetic information is therefore included in newborn screening programs (for example, for spinal muscular atrophy) and is expected to expand to an increasing number of predefined diseases, allowing identification of the disease and prevention and treatment beginning right after birth and even before initial symptoms manifest.

At the same time, improved diagnostic methods in genetic medicine—namely next generation sequencing (NGS)—make it possible to simultaneously identify multiple genes associated with different diseases that might not (yet) have resulted in any symptoms or might not even affect the person tested, but may have implications for his or her children.[1] Such predictive genetic testing can shorten the time to diagnose a disease but goes along with complex estimations of disease probability, because only a small number of diseases is actually due to a single, monogenic cause, and only few genetic constellations clearly determine a specific outcome. This means that medical communication and psychological concepts of probability and risk perception, as well as predictors of decision-making, are becoming highly relevant in this context.

The availability and affordability of genome-wide or exome-wide testing have led to more clinicians and families than ever before facing the decision of

---

[1] See, for example, M. F. Berger and E. R. Mardis, "The Emerging Clinical Relevance of Genomics in Cancer Medicine," *Nature Reviews Clinical Oncology* 15, no. 6 (2018): 353–65.

whether to use genetic tests and how to interpret the probabilistic information of the test results. As with all screening, the goal is to adjust preventive treatment or lifestyle and to increase quality of life and life expectancy. Consequently—and given the clear medical advantage of newborn screening for a number of health-limiting conditions—different countries now evaluate scenarios for genomic screening of (yet) asymptomatic newborns (gNBS). This development results in far-reaching ethical, legal, and social implications (ELSI), which need to be investigated.[2] To date, the most thoroughly studied gNBS studies with a focus on ELSI aspects are the BabySeq Project,[3] the NEXUS Project[4]—both in the United States—and the Newborn Genomes Programme in the United Kingdom. In Heidelberg, we have begun to investigate the ELSI aspects of a potential implementation of gNBS in Germany, with a focus on communication and decision processes in interaction with the necessary legal requirements and ethical implications.

In this chapter, we focus on the psychological predictors of and consequences for individuals and families during and following gNBS, namely the consequences for the family, the perception of uncertainty, and decision-making under stress.

Consequences for Individuals and Families

Genetic newborn screening is already applied as part of newborn screening in Germany for predefined conditions (for example, spinal muscular atrophy), for which early intervention can improve health or save lives. Beyond this, predictive genetic testing is possible in families with a history of a childhood-onset disorder or disorders for which preventive interventions are available.

Predictive genetic screening means that in case of a pathogenic genetic variant, there is an increased risk or susceptibility for the individual or his or her relatives to develop a specific disease. Thus, to test or not to test a newborn using gNBS as well as interpreting the results and coping with the consequences can potentially involve more than the parents and their child but also other relatives. Test results might be interpreted for individual risk reduction but also for reproductive decision-making; testing thus requires communication about intergenerational aspects of genetic disorders, family planning, and broader topics,

---

[2] L. Downie et al., "Principles of Genomic Newborn Screening Programs: A Systematic Review," *JAMA Network Open* 4, no. 7 (2021): e2114336-e2114336.

[3] I. A. Holm et al., "The BabySeq Project: Implementing Genomic Sequencing in Newborns," *BMC Pediatrics* 18, no. 1 (2018): 225.

[4] R. S. Roman et al., "Genomic Sequencing for Newborn Screening: Results of the NC NEXUS Project," *American Journal of Human Genetics* 107, no. 4 (2020): 596–611.

such as genetic determination, health images, and family roles. Theories involving concepts of family scripts, roles, and stories, such as Family Systems Theory, have been used to analyze family communication of genetic test results.[5]

In a summary of thirty-three original studies on family communication about genetic risk, M. Wiseman and colleagues identified four functions: (1) discharging responsibility for informing the family, (2) needing to gain emotional support, (3) obtaining information from the family, and (4) preventing illness through sharing the risk status. These functions were influenced by the perceived responsibility to inform, the type and quality of relationship with the persons involved, the mutation status, and personal feelings.[6]

So far, genetic counselling addresses these aspects in a nondirective way. With gNBS screening, these aspects need to be taken into account and might result in the following questions:

- How do I/we personally think about genetic determination of diseases?
- Do I/we have personal experiences in our own family history with how diseases were handled?
- Who should be involved in deciding whether to take a test?
- Who should be informed about which results?
- How would I/we handle a difficult result?

Family members might fundamentally differ in their responses to these questions. Previous research shows that females, adults, and first-degree relatives tend be informed more easily than males and second-degree or more distant relatives or young children. Regarding gNBS, this fact leads to the question of when and how to inform a child about a specific genetic condition while offering the best available care and still valuing the child's autonomy. Sharing gNBS has been discussed as potentially having negative effects, such as perceived child vulnerability, altered parent-child bonding, and self-blame and partner blame.[7]

Besides the immediate communication between parents and child, however, other genetically related family members might need to be informed, with potential consequences for their reproductive planning, health care, and insurance status. While surveys using hypothetical scenarios suggest that the majority of adults aim to receive as much information as possible, these numbers drop considerably when actual screening behavior is investigated. In her overview and

---

[5] R. MacLeod, A. Metcalfe, and M. A. Ferrer-Duch, "A Family Systems Approach to Genetic Counseling: Development of Narrative Interventions," *Journal of Genetic Counseling* 30 (2021): 22-29, https://doi.org/10.1002/jgc4.1577.

[6] M. Wiseman, C. Dancyger, and S. Michie, "Communicating Genetic Risk Information within Families: A Review," *Familial Cancer* 9, no. 4 (2010): 691-703.

[7] L. A. Frankel, S. Pereira, and A. L. McGuire, "Potential Psychosocial Risks of Sequencing Newborns," *Pediatrics* 137, Suppl. 1 (2016): S24-S29.

conceptual paper, S. H. McDaniel cites studies in which between 50 and 80 percent of individuals at risk expressed a desire to be tested, before a test was available.[8] However, when the test became widely available, only 10 to 20 percent actually sought testing. This "intention-behavior-gap" is a well-known phenomenon in behavioral medicine. It suggests that not only might there be conflicting attitudes *between* family members about genetic testing in general and gNBS in particular, but there might also be *ambivalence* within individuals and different motivations depending on age, actionability of a genetic diagnosis, the kind of disease, or whether the test is available.

In a recent qualitative study from Australia, many participants had postponed thinking about sharing results from genomic sequencing with family members and chose to wait and see whether they received actionable or severe results.[9] These findings are in line with those from an earlier study, in which relatives of individuals with informative test results were more likely to have been informed about the test results than those whose proband's test results had been uninformative.[10]

Dealing with Uncertainty

In a gNBS-scenario, with an increasing number of genes screened using NGS, there is necessarily an increase in the overall number of probability scores regarding different disorders, the frequency of identifying a variant of uncertain significance (VUS), and the number of false positives.

From established screening and diagnostic programs, there is research on how individuals process probabilistic information and uncertainty in a medical context, and how parents handle false positives in newborn screening. In these studies, besides the actual testing rate, outcome variables included emotional responses, health literacy and knowledge, behavioral responses, and disease related quality of life.

---

[8] S. H. McDaniel, "The Psychotherapy of Genetics," *Family Process* 44, no. 1 (2005): 25-44.

[9] A. K. Smit et al., "Family Communication about Genomic Sequencing: A Qualitative Study with Cancer Patients and Relatives," *Patient Education and Counseling* 104, no. 5 (2021): 944-52.

[10] M. B. Daly et al., "Communicating Genetic Test Results within the Family: Is It Lost in Translation? A Survey of Relatives in the Randomized Six-Step Study," *Familial Cancer* 15, no. 4 (2016): 697-706.

Probability Scores

By themselves, a high number of different *probability scores* are difficult to assess regarding implications for immediate behavior or even more far-reaching consequences, such as family planning. Imagine the scenario that gNBS results suggest a 40 percent risk of developing breast cancer, a 30 percent risk of developing ovarian cancer, and a 25 percent risk of developing a life-threatening cardiac condition. How parents process these different probability scores depends on their individual representation of numerical risk in combination with the emotional content of each health outcome. This combination in part explains whether individuals take concrete follow-up steps or not.

Comprehension of numerical risk-and-benefit information plays an important role in whether individuals show intentions to screen for diseases and how they interpret the results.[11] Numerical and risk literacy can be trained, and educational material has been designed to inform parents about the risks and benefits of current newborn screening programs. These, however, need substantial adaptation, because parallel testing of multiple genetic constellations and the higher number of diseases screened for will increase the number of single probability scores.

Individual personality traits and coping styles can explain in part why some people use genetic testing while others rely on their right not to know. Among such coping styles are the tendency to show monitoring behavior (that is, scanning for and amplifying threatening cues) in contrast to blunting behavior (minimizing or avoiding threatening cues). Moreover, a person's own family history and emotionally driven memories, as well as visually presented material rather than verbatim information, seem to influence how individuals interpret the "gist" of information provided to them.[12]

Research from genetic newborn screening for single predefined diseases suggests that the parents' (mostly the mother's) perception of risk and their individual well-being (as indicated through anxiety and depression levels) or behavior depend, among other things, on prenatal mental health, education, social background, living situation, and age of the child at the time of the screening.[13]

---

[11] D. Petrova et al., "To Screen or Not to Screen: What Factors Influence Complex Screening Decisions?," *Journal of Experimental Psychology: Applied* 22, no. 2 (2016): 247–60.

[12] V. F. Reyna, "A Theory of Medical Decision Making and Health: Fuzzy Trace Theory," *Medical Decision Making* 28, no. 6 (2008): 850–65.

[13] For discussion, see N. Dikow et al.,"From Newborn Screening to Genomic Medicine: Challenges and Suggestions on How to Incorporate Genomic Newborn Screening in Public Health Programs," *Medizinische Genetik* 34, no. 1 (2022): 13–20.

False Positives

False positives can be part of the measurement procedure; these are out-of-range results that are not confirmed by a repeat measurement. Generally, these results are not laboratory mistakes but rather are transient findings or indications of variant or carrier status.[14] In newborn screening, false positives can substantially impair the parents' well-being and mental health. In an overview, J. Hewlett and S. E. Waisbren report that eight out of nine original studies found increased parental anxiety and/or depression after a false positive result, even after the repeat test was normal.[15] Moreover, false positive test results can increase parental stress, as suggested from studies using the Parenting Stress Index (PSI). In a large study, mothers in the false positive group screened significantly higher in the PSI than mothers in the normal screened group.[16]

Some of the original studies also reported long-term effects on parental perception of their infant's health, including increased hospitalizations for the child. These results suggest that false positives can have far-reaching consequences for health perception within a family and parent-child interactions, and that parents need to be informed about the relative number of false positives and provided with informational brochures and in-person information on concrete next steps to take after an initial positive test result, on the general percentage of false positives, and on the possible outcomes of repeat tests.

Notably, stress levels associated with false positives could be buffered when the results of a repeat screen were communicated in person instead of by telephone or letter.[17] It seems reasonable that reassuring results from the repeat test appear "more real" when communicated personally in comparison to a phone call or a letter. In addition, our own research as well as that of others suggest that real-life social contact can buffer stress levels via the genuine perception of social integration and support and independently of the content communicated.[18] This suggests that in screening programs where false results are probable, standard procedures should be implemented to invite parents back and inform them about the repeat-testing results in person.

---

[14] W. J. Tu et al., "Psychological Effects of False-Positive Results in Expanded Newborn Screening in China," *PloS One* 7, no. 4 (2012): e36235.

[15] J. Hewlett and S. E. Waisbren, "A Review of the Psychosocial Effects of False-Positivve Results on Parents and Current Communication Practices in Newborn Screening," *Journal of Inherited Metabolic Disease* 29, no. 5 (2006): 677–82.

[16] S. E. Waisbren et al., "Effect of Expanded Newborn Screening for Biochemical Genetic Disorders on Child Outcomes and Parental Stress," *JAMA* 290, no. 19 (2003): 2564–72.

[17] Ibid.

[18] B. Ditzen and M. Heinrichs, "Psychobiology of Social Support: The Social Dimension of Stress Burffering," *Restorative Neurology and Neuroscience* 32, no. 1 (2014): 149–62.

Variants of Uncertain Significance

Variants of uncertain significance (VUS) are variants in genes associated with disease risk, where evidence is insufficient to conclude whether they are pathogenic or a rather benign polymorphism (that is, an ambiguous result).[19] Thus, the consequences of VUS are challenging to communicate and can result in uncertainty in clinicians and patients alike.[20] While the clinician's communicating of uncertainty can have beneficial effects by enhancing patient autonomy and realistic expectations, it can also overwhelm patients and increase their worries.[21]

In reviewing twenty-four original studies, N. M. Medendorp and colleagues report that counselees often interpret VUS incorrectly, although this was not systematically associated with improved or impaired positive affect or quality of life.[22] As the authors discuss, the counselees' personality and uncertainty tolerance as a trait might affect how they perceive communication of VUS and how this perception affects their adaptation to the results. It might be assumed that communicating VUS has a negative impact on the perception of the clinician's competence and thereby increases distress, although to our knowledge this has not been investigated yet.

Actionability

Using five different dimensions to evaluate a genetic variant's impact on an outcome, J. S. Berg and colleagues developed a "semiquantitative metric" of actionability.[23] These dimensions included (1) severity, (2) likelihood, (3) efficacy of intervention, (4) burden of intervention, and (5) knowledge base. This metric

---

[19] H. Duzkale et al., "A Systematic Approach to Assessing the Clinical Significance of Genetic Variants," *Clinical Genetics* 84, no. 5 (Nov. 2013): 453–63, doi: 10.1111/cge.12257. PMID: 24033266; PMCID: PMC3995020.

[20] L. P. Spees et al., "Involving Patients and Their Families in Deciding to Use Next Generation Sequencing: Results from a Nationally Representative Survey of U.S. Oncologists," *Patient Education and Counseling* 104, no. 1 (2021): 33–39.

[21] N. M. Medendorp et al., "The Impact of Communicating Uncertain Test Results in Cancer Genetic Counseling: A Systematic Mixed Studies Review," *Patient Education and Counseling* 103, no. 9 (2020): 1692–708.

[22] Ibid.

[23] J. S. Berg et al., "A Semiquantitative Metric for Evaluating Clinical Actionability of Incidental or Secondary Findings from Genome-Scale Sequencing," *Genetics in Medicine* 18, no. 5 (2016): 467–75.

might serve as tool to guide communication about whether, when, and with whom to share genetic findings.

Actionability can also help to structure the screening process from the *clinician's perspective*. However, from the *patient's or the parents' perspective*, both trait and state characteristics predict how individuals will handle probabilistic information and medical uncertainty and consider relevant benefits, harms, risks, and limitations when making health-relevant decisions. Different psychological models cover these aspects, with special emphasis on emotional involvement, cognitive skills, and attitudes, as well as comprehension of the complex (numerical) information involved.[24]

The Mental Models Approach to Risk Communication (MMARC) has been developed to acknowledge that an individual's mental representation of a concept is a combination of personal experiences and statistical and/or verbatim information, and thus not always based on accurate information.[25] This finding resonates with the Fuzzy Trace Theory, which suggests that exemplary and visually represented memories determine how complex information is processed.[26] Both theories become relevant, and their parameters supposedly interact with momentary stress levels in predicting decision making.

Overall predictive genetic testing may have less distressing consequences than originally anticipated.[27] However, parents might be differently affected depending on their level of engagement with the child, their gender and social role, individual values, and whether they themselves are the carrier of a critical mutation or not. This requires *dyadic decision-making*, a task that is well known in family counseling and psychotherapy but less intensely studied in the context of somatic medicine.

Dyadic Decision-Making

The decision in favor of or against gNBS involves both parents and is a dyadic decision. Therefore, dyadic decision models can help to identify parameters that predict (a) whether couples decide to use genomic testing and (b) if so, how they wish the results to be communicated.

Previous research on reproductive genetic testing or screening suggests that couples showed high agreement in psychological variables, such as risk and

---

[24] For an overview and discussion, see Petrova et al., "To Screen or Not to Screen."
[25] M. G. Morgan et al., *Risk Communication: A Mental Models Approach* (Cambridge: Cambridge University Press, 2002).
[26] Reyna, "A Theory of Medical Decision Making and Health: Fuzzy Trace Theory."
[27] C. Lerman et al., "Genetic Testing: Psychological Aspects and Implications," *Journal of Consulting and Clinical Psychology* 70, no. 3 (2022): 784–97.

benefit perceptions about genetic variant status, attitudes about reproductive testing, genetic stigma beliefs, or affect relating to receiving the test results. There was also dyadic correlation in the couples' tendency to share the test results with family members. However, relatively few dyadic predictors were found to explain these correlations; those predictors were communication quality, confidence in the partner's ability to cope with the test results, and a stronger parenting alliance.[28]

With regard to gNBS, parental interest was shown to be independent of the parents' age, gender, ethnicity, level of education, or family history of a genetic disease, although about a quarter of couples in which both partners were surveyed were discordant in their attitudes toward performing gNBS in their own child.[29] In couples therapy, communication methods have been developed to help both partners identify and communicate about difficult, ambivalent, and discrepant topics in their relationship.[30] These methods include guided and structured dialogue sequences, in which each partner expresses interpretations, feelings, and ideas about future outcomes in predefined roles. Such interventions from clinical psychology might be of use to structure genetic counseling in an gNBS setting[31] and help parents identify and express their individual values with the goal of reaching concordant decisions.

Decision Aids

Not only patients but also clinicians describe barriers to using genomic screening instruments. In a recent survey, 59 percent of oncologists reported barriers to involving patients in the decision-making process for use of next-generation sequencing, most of them citing a lack of educational material and difficulties getting patients to understand the results and treatment options in the limited time available.[32] This suggests that educational material, standard decision tools, and communication training might help overcome such barriers.

---

[28] W. K. Law et al., Decision-Making about Genetic Health Information among Family Dyads: A Systematic Literature Review," *Health Psychology Review* 16, no 3 (2022): 412–29.

[29] S. E. Waisbren et al., "Parents Are Interested in Newborn Genomic Testing during the Early Postpartum Period," *Genetics in Medicine* 17, no. 6 (2015): 501–04.

[30] B. Silliman et al., "Preventive Interventions for Couples," in *Family Psychology: Science-Based Interventions*, ed. H. A. Liddle et al., 123–146 (Washington, DC: American Psychological Association, 2002), https://doi.org/10.1037/10438-007.

[31] McDaniel, "The Psychotherapy of Genetics."

[32] Spees et al., "Involving Patients and Their Families in Deciding to Use Next Generation Sequencing."

Shared decision-making (SDM) describes a model of medical communication that involves the patient's values and attitudes and the pros and cons of a decision. More recently, SDM has been translated to genetic counseling. A recent study, although small, observed that SDM levels reduce anxiety or decisional conflict in individuals during genetic counseling.[33] SDM might, indeed, help improve dyadic agreement in parents who decide about gNBS. One important aspect is that SDM relies on the possibility of deferring the decision and making follow-up appointments. This might help in discussing and restructuring pros and cons, reducing stress levels, improving cognitive flexibility, and, thereby, reducing decisional conflict in the long term.

A large number of interventions to improve decision-making in genetic medicine have been developed and, overall, have resulted in improved knowledge-related, behavior-related, and/or well-being-related outcomes in patients.[34] To ease decision-making in a complex and value-based medical context, decision aids have been developed which, in a structured communication procedure, try to:
- provide information in sufficient detail;
- couch probabilities of outcomes in an unbiased and understandable way; and
- include tools to help patients elaborate on and express their values.

International Patient Decision Aid Standards (IPDAS) have been defined and focus on the development process of such decision aids. The IPDAS are publicly available online.[35] In the U.S.-based NEXUS project, a decision aid was developed for gNBS.[36] Initial results from qualitative interviews with thirty-three couples suggest that more than 90 percent of participants (sixty out of sixty-six) said they would choose gNBS if it was offered for their newborn, and they saw the possibility of early intervention as a major benefit in genomic screening. They also saw a potential in gNBS to prepare physically, financially, and emotionally for the potential onset of disease. However, the study participants also expressed some worries anticipating the worst-case scenario in case of a positive screening or fears of stigma. Overall, participants were more likely to choose to

---

[33] P. H. Birch et al., "Assessing Shared Decision-Making Clinical Behaviors among Genetic Counsellors," *Journal of Genetic Counseling* 28, no. 8 (2018): doi https://doi.org/10.1007/s10897-018-0285-x.

[34] F. Legare et al., "Improving Decision Making about Genetic Testing in the Clinic: An Overview of Effective Knowledge Translation Interventions," *PloS One* 11, no. 3 (2016): e0150123.

[35] http://www.ipdas.ohri.ca/.

[36] M. A. Lewis et al., "Supporting Parental Decisions about Genomic Sequencing for Newborn Screening: The NC NEXUS Decision Aid," *Pediatrics* 137, Suppl. 1 (2016): S16–23.

learn test results for actionable rather than nonactionable diseases, and diseases with a childhood onset rather than an adult onset.

Information Processing and Decision-Making under Stress

In genetic counseling of newborn screening, when health or even survival of the child is at stake, stress levels can be high, and the processing and memory of important information might be impaired.[37] With regard to gNBS, this becomes particularly relevant in the sharing of complex information and probability predictions, which demand decisions that can have an impact not only on the child's immediate health but also on other family members' health decisions.[38]

On a neural level in the brain, decisions made under risk conditions evoke activities in the dorsolateral prefrontal cortex, the ventral prefrontal cortex, the anterior cingulate gyrus, the anterior cingulate cortex, the orbitofrontal cortex, and the parietal cortex. More emotional-intuitive decisions rely on limbic and basal ganglia activation, which can also trigger a faster response.[39] Under stress conditions, a switch from top-down prefrontal modulation to faster bottom-up processes has been suggested, based on animal and human research.[40] In line with this, psychobiological stress has been shown to alter information processing and behavior, depending on the level of central nervous system activation of mineralocorticoid and glucocorticoid receptors.[41] This means, that under high-stress conditions, individuals' capability to process complex numerical information and to decide in a well-balanced and rational way might be impaired. Rather, decisions might be based on emotional representations of earlier experiences and according to routine-behavioral patterns.

In one study, parents who were asked about hypothetical genomic testing of their newborn reported lower interest in testing when they had a newborn with

---

[37] C. P. Schaaf, S. Kölker, and G. F. Hoffmann, "Genomic Newborn Screening: Proposal of a Two-Stage Approach," *Journal of Inherited Metabolic Disease* 44, no. 3 (May 2021): 518–20, doi: 10.1002/jimd.12381.

[38] C. P. Schaaf, "Genetic Counseling and the Role of Genetic Counselors in the United States," *Medizinische Genetik* 33, no. 1 (2021): 29–34.

[39] K. Starcke and M. Brand, "Decision Making under Stress: A Selective Review," *Neuroscience & Biobehavioral Reviews* 36, no. 4 (2012): 1228–48.

[40] A. F. Arnsten, "Stress Signalling Pathways That Impair Prefrontal Cortex Structure and Function," *Nature Reviews Neuroscience*, 10, no. 6 (2009): 410–22.

[41] R. M. Sapolsky, "Stress and the Brain: Individual Variability and Inverted-U," *Nature Neuroscience* 18, no. 10 (2015): 1344–46.

health concerns.[42] These results might seem counterintuitive at first but could be interpreted in terms of the parents' stress-induced wish to avoid new or more complex information on the health condition of their child or a hereditary component of this condition. According to the authors of the study, "It is possible that parents who reported that their child had a health concern were more stressed and less interested in genetic testing because of its potential to increase their emotional distress."[43]

In two ongoing studies, we currently investigate (a) how psychobiological stress (as assessed via self-report and stress-sensitive cortisol levels) affects memory in the presentation of different diagnoses (including genetic diagnoses) in standard scenarios in healthy individuals and (b) whether preprocessing of information, as presented in standard educational videos, can buffer subjective stress levels during genetic counseling in patients. To our knowledge, it is unclear how acute stress might affect parents' decisions to take up gNBS, to understand its results, or to communicate the results with family members. Moreover, on a more precise level, it would be relevant to investigate whether stress levels influence the perception of the "gist" of health-relevant information[44] when information is shared following gNBS.

Summary and Outlook

While NGS and gNBS represent enormous advances in genetic diagnostic testing and make screening of life-threatening or debilitating diseases possible at an early moment in life, the resulting complex and probabilistic data can be difficult to manage for the families involved.

In an ongoing interdisciplinary project (led by Prof. Dr. Eva C. Winkler), we are currently beginning to investigate the medical, ethical, legal, and psychological perspective on genome-wide sequencing technology for newborn screening. In a qualitative study including focus groups and a quantitative part on (prospective) parents' preferences and values, we aim to determine the parents' and patients' perspectives on the potentials but also the risks of genomic newborn screening. Future research might aim to integrate data from neurobiological stress research into dyadic decision models and emotion-focused decision models, such as the fuzzy trace theory in the context of gNBS.

In the actual context of genetic counseling, shared decision-making (SDM) and guided communication based on tools from couple counseling might be used to help parents elaborate on their own values and ambivalences and reduce mo-

---

[42] Waisbren et al., "Parents Are Interested in Newborn Genomic Testing."
[43] Ibid., 502.
[44] Reyna, "A Theory of Medical Decision Making and Health."

mentary stress levels. Beyond this, from international and ongoing gNBS studies, there are initial interventions and tools available with the aim to educate, increase health literacy, reduce stress levels, and improve parental agreement with potential long-term benefits for the families involved.

Part Four: Health Care: History, Education, Practice

On the History of the Nursing Ethos in Germany

Karen Nolte

The nursing profession is currently very present in the public perception because of its important role in coping with the COVID-19 pandemic over the past three years. The pandemic has brought even more attention to the already obvious nursing crisis, not least because nurses have spoken out on social media, on talk shows, and as authors of books. In the following, I offer, on one hand, insight into the history of the nursing ethos, and on the other hand I show how the nursing emergency has influenced the work of nurses since the late 1950 s, and how nurses perceived the dehumanization in health care due to increasing rationalization and economization.

The Nursing Ethos in Germany

In this first section, I identify early normative ideas about the ideal nurse. What made a good nurse? How was a nurse supposed to behave?

Doctors in Germany made the first efforts to systematically train nurses by setting up so-called schools for orderlies. In 1782, the Mannheim physician Franz Anton May (1742–1814) published a book entitled *Instruction for Orderlies*.[1] In contrast to the supposedly "chatty" and "nosy" women in nursing, the orderlies trained in the doctor's schools were to be educated to conscientiously follow medical regulations.

In 1832, the Berlin surgeon Johann Friedrich Dieffenbach (1792–1847), in his *Instructions for Nursing* (*Anleitung zur Krankenwartung*), described the essential qualities of nurses as those that were more characteristic of women, namely cleanliness and virtue. On the other hand, Dieffenbach's willingness to provide selfless care did not yet have gender-specific connotations. Prudence, vigilance, and attentiveness characterized a good orderly just as much as the ability to con-

---

[1] Franz Anton May, *Unterricht für Krankenwärter zum Gebrauch öffentlicher Vorlesungen* (Mannheim: Schwanische Buchhandlung, 1782).

scientiously carry out medical orders and "literally" what he was ordered to do by the doctor.²

While doctors around 1800 sought to establish nursing as a medical auxiliary activity, the pastor Theodor Fliedner (1800–1864) pursued a different goal by founding the first deaconess institute in Kaiserswerth, near Düsseldorf. There, young women were trained as nurses to care for the sick in poor neighborhoods. The Protestant bourgeoisie regretted that people from the urban proletariat in particular had lost their Christian faith. They saw their task in the "inner mission," that is, the rechristianization of the unbelieving poor. Poverty was attributed causally to illness, and illness was interpreted as a consequence of unbelief and a sinful way of life. Consequently, good training in nursing should serve to combat illness as well as poverty, including spiritual poverty. Therefore, Fliedner sent his nurses to the poor quarters and hospitals that cared mainly for poor people, in order to gain access to their souls through nursing.³

What should the ideal Protestant nurse be like? Essential qualities are formulated in a handwritten teaching manuscript from Kaiserswerth: attentiveness, presence of mind, cold-bloodedness without harshness or indifference, mildness ... without sensibility, cheerfulness in the right sense, discretion, truthfulness, punctuality, and agreeableness. Here we find qualities that did not have gender-specific connotations.⁴ The nursing ethos can be seen in the manuscript on the training of deaconesses: A nurse could not learn too much. She should also learn medical tasks that she could perform when the doctor was not available. Since she was committed to the principle of self-denial, there was hardly any danger of her using her knowledge to take the place of the doctor. The house and service regulations state that the nursing deaconess should follow the "prescriptions of the family doctor with regard to medicine, bandaging, care and diet of the sick punctually and without protest."⁵ In fact, this obedience was clearly limited to bodily care—the care of the soul was an area of competence in which doctors were not granted any authority to issue directives. With the catalogue of self-examination questions, deaconesses were to internalize the nursing ethos of the community daily. Central authorities for deaconesses were the superior cou-

---

2   Johann Friedrich Dieffenbach, *Anleitung zur Krankenwartung* (Berlin: Verlag von August Hirschwald, 1832).
3   Karen Nolte, "Protestant Nursing Care in Germany in the 19th Century—Concepts and Social Practice," in *Handbook for the Global History of Nursing, London*, ed. Patricia D'Antonio, Julie Fairman, and Jean Whelan (London: Routledge, 2013), 167–82.
4   Theodor Fliedner, *Medicinischer Cursus* (1850), Heft 3, § 2, Archive of the Fliedner Kulturstiftung Kaiserswerth (AFKSK).
5   Theodor Fliedner, *Haus- und Dienst-Anweisung für die Diakonissen und Probeschwester in der Diakonissen-Anstalt zu Kaiserwerth* (1852), § 4, i 3, Archive of the Fliedner Kulturstiftung Kaiserswerth (AFKSK).

ple of the deaconess community and God, who is always mentioned by the deaconesses in their letters as the "heavenly physician," who alone determined whether a sick person could be healed.

A glance at the *Notes on Nursing* published by Florence Nightingale (1820–1910) in 1860 shows what standards the famous British reformer of nursing applied to a "good nurse": she deliberately formulated a secular nursing ethos.[6] After her visit to Kaiserswerth in 1849, Nightingale was critical of the importance of piety in the training and practice in nursing there. She created a system of training that was distinct from the religious sisterhood. According to Nightingale, a "good nurse" was a person who acted professionally and who placed the greatest value on the close observation of the patients entrusted to her care. However, the nurse had to feel a vocation to nursing, since without this vocation she could not meet the needs of the sick despite thorough training in nursing. Nightingale argued against the widespread view that nurses should be "devoted and obedient"—attributes appropriate for a horse, but not for a nurse. In contrast, she speaks of "intelligent obedience," where the nurse should assess for herself how sensible it is to implement an order. This contextual obedience to the doctor and matron is similar to the understanding that can be found in normative texts in Kaiserswerth. In the system developed by Nightingale, too, the "head nurses" and, in the last instance, the lady superintendent of nurses, who came from the upper class, represented the essential authorities to whom the nurses' actions were related.[7]

Nightingale objected to the ever-emphasized qualities of a nurse to be "sober, honest, and chaste." These qualities applied to any woman but did not describe the specific requirements of a nurse. The ideal qualities described for Kaiserswerth nurses as "compassion without sentimentality" and "cold-bloodedness without indifference" are bundled by Nightingale under the term "countenance," with which nurses were to face despair and unpleasant symptoms of illness.

While in denominational nursing the activity was understood as a vocation in the religious sense, Florence Nightingale defined nursing as a professional activity already in the nineteenth century. In Great Britain and in the countries influenced by the British nursing system, nursing was therefore professionalized at an early stage.

The Nightingale system was taken up by only a few nursing schools in Germany—for example, by the Berlin physician Rudolf Virchow, who around 1900 called for professional training in nursing that would combine the sacrificial na-

---

[6] Florence Nightingale, *Notes on Nursing: What It Is, and What It Is Not* (New York: D. Appleton, 1860).
[7] Ibid.

ture of Christian nurses with scientific training led by doctors.[8] Another example is the Clementinenstiftung (Clementine's Foundation) in Hanover, which trained nurses based on the Nightingale System and was run by the activist of the bourgeois women's movement Olga Freiin von Lützerode (1836-1917). Agnes Karll (1868-1927), the later cofounder of the Professional Organization of Nurses in Germany, had completed her training there. What was special about the training in Hanover was that the student nurses were taught by physicians both practically in the clinic and theoretically. The focus was therefore on delivering medical knowledge.[9]

The professional association of nurses in Germany—also called the Agnes Karll Association—was largely shaped by Karll and aimed to reconcile elements of the denominational sisterhoods with "modern life" and a beginning professional understanding of nursing. The professional title "sister" was still chosen, and the nursing ethos formulated nursing as "serving love." Heartfelt mercy and intimate compassion for the sick, kindness, humility, gentleness, patience, discipline, and self-control were the central qualities a nurse should have. The motto of the professional organization was, "Ich diene!" (I serve!) On one hand, this motto tied in with the Christian tradition of nursing as a service of love—the motto of the Kaiserswerth deaconesses was "Dienen will ich" (I will serve)—and, on the other hand, the shortened verb referred to military "serving," or service to the fatherland. With its nursing ethos, the professional organization referred to the concept of "spiritual motherliness" of the bourgeois women's movement, which assumed that the "innate motherly love" of all women could be lived out in the field of social work as an alternative to bodily motherhood. Nursing was to be understood as a profession, which was expressed through demands for state-recognized training and for a limit on working hours. It was also an expression of limited working hours that the Agnes Karll sisters were able to take off their sisterly uniforms at the end of their service, while deaconesses had to wear their uniforms at all times in public, thus demonstrating that they were always on duty. Free time, as opposed to working time, was thus an expression of a professional self-image of the sisters from the Agnes Karll Association.[10]

In 1907, one-year training in state-recognized nursing schools was introduced in most German states. However, Agnes Karll had already called for three

---

[8] Eduard Seidler and Karl-Heinz Leven, *Geschichte der Medizin und der Krankenpflege*, 7th edition (Stuttgart, Kohlhammer, 2003), 224-25.

[9] Traudel Weber-Reich, *"Wir sind die Pionierinnen der Pflege ..."*: *Krankenschwestern und ihre Pflegestätten im 19. Jahrhundert am Beispiel Göttingen* (Bern: Huber, 2003).

[10] Brigitte Kerchner, *Beruf und Geschlecht: Frauenberufsverbände in Deutschland 1848-1908* (Göttingen: Vandenhoeck & Ruprecht, 1992), 170-86.

years of training around 1900—a demand that was not to be implemented until the Nursing Act of 1965.[11]

In 1911, before World War I, Anna von Zimmermann, superior of the Sisterhood of the Red Cross, published her book *Was heißt Schwester Sein?* (What does it mean to be a nurse?), in which she formulated the basics of the professional ethos for nurses of the Sisterhood of the Red Cross.[12] This document, which appeared in several editions, formulated a nursing ethos that was to be influential for the self-image of nurses until well into the twentieth century. Zimmermann described nursing not as a profession but as an "activity of love," because "it is not a trade, it should be a work of love, not a job for personal gain, but for the sake of God and others, for the sake of a great cause. It is not a craft, it should be a work of love, selfless, faithful service. What is demanded of a sister in terms of physical effort, in terms of surrender of all personal life demands, in terms of sacrifice, in terms of self-conquest, cannot be paid for."[13]

Zimmerman clearly defined nursing as an assistant medical activity. The nurse had to be aware of her limits, the greater her skills became. Her position must be "as a helper next to the doctor." The doctor was the one who always determined the limits of her services.[14] The Sisterhoods of the German Red Cross had originated in 1864 as various organizations whose decentralized associations were to train and organize nurses to care for the war-wounded. With their hierarchical organization, they followed the structures of the military. Anna von Zimmermann therefore formulated the relationship between doctor and nurses accordingly, with military metaphors:

> Like a commander with his troops, the doctor works with his nurses, who are subordinate to him. Without a commander, the work of the troops is aimless; without troops, the work of the commander is unsuccessful. Both are important and yet separate areas, between which obedience forms the connecting link. ... The commander is the doctor, his adjutant the leading ward nurse, the troops the learning, teaching, and probationary nurses who must serve from the ground up in order to be able to teach themselves later. Only those who have learned to subordinate, to submit, and to serve will be able to govern.[15]

---

[11] Sylvelyn Hähner-Rombach, "Aus- und Weiterbildung in der Krankenpflege in der Bundesrepublik Deutschland nach 1945," in *Entwicklungen in der Krankenpflege und in anderen Gesundheitsberufen nach 1945. Ein Lehr- und Studienbuch*, ed. Sylvelyn Hähner-Rombach and Pierre Pfütsch (Frankfurt am Main: Mabuse-Verlag, 2018), 146–94; and Seidler and Leven, *Geschichte der Medizin und der Krankenpflege*, 228.

[12] Anna von Zimmermann, *Was heißt Schwester Sein? Beiträge zur ethischen Berufsbezeichnung* (Berlin: Springer, 1911). The translation was done by the author of this article.

[13] Ibid., 8.

[14] Ibid., 22.

[15] Ibid., 37.

Zimmermann swore her sisters to unconditional obedience to the doctor. Even a nurse with much professional experience should not be allowed under any circumstances to question the orders of a young, inexperienced doctor. A nurse was allowed to cross the line into the doctor's area of competence only if an emergency arose and a doctor was not available.

Recall Nightingale's remarks. In Zimmermann's writing we find an explicit reference to Nightingale's "intelligent obedience," but the principle of obedience between doctors and nurses was very strongly emphasized. Zimmermann elevated unconditional obedience and submission to the basic principle of the relationship between nurses and doctors, which was not to be questioned at all. For example, she said that an experienced nurse may not disagree with an inexperienced young physician even if her experience led her to the conclusion that the physician was making an erratic order. Nightingale, on the other hand, also addressed physicians with the demand to recognize the competences of experienced nurses and to treat them respectfully.

Physicians formulated their ideas of an obedient, hardworking, and humble nurse in the nursing textbooks they wrote in great numbers. But it is rare to find texts in which physicians reflected on their own behavior toward nurses. Albert Moll published in 1901 his *Ärztliche Ethik* (Ethics for doctors) and held the opinion that it could only be beneficial for a young doctor if he learned in his ethical training to administer medicine, or to put a bedpan under the patient, as well as acquiring nursing skills, such as lifting and transferring a patient to a different bed. Moll argued for a nursing internship for medical students so that they would gain a deeper understanding of the nursing profession. Moll's relationship to nurses was probably not representative for his profession, as there were a number of authors of nursing books who rather confirmed Zimmermann's idea of the doctor-nurse relationship.[16]

Nursing Shortage, Rationalization, Savings—and Criticism

Until well into the twentieth century, nursing in Germany was organized in sisterhoods, most of which were influenced by denominations. Nursing was understood by both the Christian and the increasingly founded secular sisterhoods as a loving service, that is, a decidedly nonprofessional understanding prevailed. Since women saw themselves committed to nursing with their entire person, their work was naturally perceived as a cost-effective resource. In the 1950 s, this life and work model of nursing came into crisis, as fewer and fewer young

---

[16] Albert Moll, *Ärztliche Ethik. Die Pflichten des Arztes in allen Beziehungen seiner Thätigkeit* (Stuttgart: Enke, 1902).

women were willing to give up a private life and family.[17] The result was a dramatic shortage of new recruits into the traditional nurses' associations.

Parallel to this development, the hospital system in West Germany was massively expanded, and the number of hospital beds increased enormously. In order to react to the increased shortage of skilled workers and the simultaneous decline in interest in the nursing profession, not only were many new nursing schools opened, but also the first attempts were made to recruit nursing staff from the southern European countries of Greece, Italy, and Spain. While in Germany a two-year, predominantly practice-oriented nursing training with an additional compulsory internship of one year was still common until 1965, nurses from the southern European countries were already academically trained at that time and therefore difficult to recruit for the German labor market.[18] These measures could therefore not effectively combat the "nurse shortage" (*Schwesternnot*). The dwindling number of qualified nurses already led to working conditions in the 1950 s that were perceived as crisis-ridden, even by sisterhoods that advocated selflessness and a strong work ethic. A 1951 article written by a doctor criticized hospital managers for exploiting nurses' altruism too economically:

> It is the noblest task of the nurse to create a soothing atmosphere in the sick rooms, and this means for her a criterion of her ability and her vocation. ... Her selfless joyful service to the sick means for her the fulfillment of a womanly and maternal existence, to which personal economic securities are of secondary importance. It is as much a sign of ignorance as it is of senseless mercantilism on the part of many hospital owners to exploit this basic attitude of the nurses for their own benefit, to exploit their labor through excessive working hours, inferior pay, sometimes even today inadequate food, inadequate accommodation, in short through intolerable personal working conditions, and to turn hospitals into health factories.[19]

The term "health factory" here initially alludes only to the exploitation or even "consumption" of the labor of selfless nurses. The nurses are still attributed a nursing ethos, according to which their work was seen as a loving service for the sick, in which the desire for appropriate payment was not in the foreground. Nevertheless, the increasingly economic orientation of hospital management

---

[17] Susanne Kreutzer, *Vom "Liebesdienst" zum modernen Frauenberuf. Die Reform der Krankenpflege nach 1945.* (Frankfurt am Main: Campus Verlag, 2005).

[18] Susanne Kreutzer, "Der Pflegenotstand der 1960er Jahre. Arbeitsalltag, Krisenwahrnehmung und Reformen," in *Pflege. Praxis - Geschichte - Politik*, ed. Bundeszentrale für politische Bildung (Bonn: APuZ, 2020), 144–55.

[19] Buurmann, "Gedanken zur Überforderung der Krankenschwestern," *Deutsche Schwesternzeitung* 4, no. 1 (1951): 4–6, at 5. Translation by the author of this article.

and the exploitation of nurses' selfless attitude is criticized. In fact, already at that time, all actors in health policy were aware that hospital treatment costs could not be financed by health-insurance contributions alone, but a solution had not yet been found. Attempts to reduce the costs of health care failed because of the resistance of general practitioners. Since 1954, the costs of hospital treatment were to be covered only to a small extent by health-insurance funds and additionally by the municipalities. However, hospital expenses could not be financed by the municipalities to cover costs, which led to successively increasing deficits in hospital budgets.[20]

In order to make the nursing profession more attractive for young German women in the long term, its framework conditions had to be changed. The aim was to make nursing more professional in order to make it compatible with marriage and family in the future. In 1961, the obligation to pay board and lodging in nursing was abolished, and soon afterward the possibility of part-time work was granted. In addition, weekly working hours were gradually reduced: in 1956 to fifty-four hours, in 1958 to fifty-one hours, and from 1960 the forty-eight-hour week applied in municipal hospitals. However, with the reduction in working hours, the need for qualified nursing staff grew at the same time, which further aggravated the nurse shortage in the course of the 1960 s. At the same time, the economic situation in the hospital sector came to a head thanks to a rising cost trend with a simultaneous drop in health-insurance contributions; the latter was caused by rising unemployment as a result of the economic downturn caused by the oil crisis. In 1974, discourse on costs became dominant in health policy.[21]

In Heidelberg at that time, nurses demanded codetermination in the distribution of the increasingly scarce resources in the hospital. In June 1971, together with students from the Heidelberg nursing school and medical students, they demonstrated against the hospital regulations, which they held responsible for the unequal distribution of funds and equipment in the hospital, under the slogan "Against health care in the service of capital—For health care in the service of the people." The daily press reported that totally "overworked nursing staff ... were no longer able to give patients the care they needed," while in private wards chief physicians were well paid for treatment.[22]

---

[20] Robin Mohan, *Die Ökonomisierung des Krankenhauses* (Bielefeld: transcript, 2019), 154–57.

[21] Jürgen Wasem, "Zur Entwicklung von Kostendämpfungspolitik und Strukturreformen im deutschen Gesundheitswesen," *Zeitschrift für Medizinische Ethik* 66, no. 2 (2020): 141–52, at 142.

[22] Rasch, "Mit Schwesternhäubchen zum Protestmarsch. Demonstration gegen die geplante Klinikordnung/Forderung: 'Entmachtet die Halbgötter in Weiß,'" *Heidelberger Tageblatt*, Jun. 12, 1971.

The Arbeitskreis Krankenhaus (Working Group Hospital) firmly criticized in a flyer: "The distribution of the budget funds, which are too low anyway, continues to be made solely by hospital bosses and the administrative director, that is, nurses, orderlies, assistants, who through their daily work on the wards know very well what is needed, remain excluded from any co-decision."[23]

Furthermore, "wrong decisions" and the "strict hierarchy in the hospital" were criticized for leading to a "bad working atmosphere" and being responsible for the "miserable working conditions" and the "lack of personnel." The fact that patient care suffered as a result was reported daily in the "press, radio and television" and experienced by patients themselves. Obviously, nurses were encouraged by the politicized climate of the new social movements, such as the student movement in Heidelberg, to publicly and loudly point out grievances and social injustices at the university hospital and to demand their codetermination. Nurses also demonstrated elsewhere against the steadily worsening working conditions in hospitals as a result of cost-cutting measures, for example in Frankfurt am Main in September 1970.[24] Meanwhile, the nursing shortage in Heidelberg came to a head, forcing the complete closure of a ward in the Surgical Clinic at Heidelberg University due to a shortage of nursing staff.[25]

In 1975, functional nursing was introduced in West German hospitals. This was an essential measure to rationalize nursing and was intended to increase efficiency in nursing through staff reductions and job cuts. Nursing tasks were now carried out according to Taylorist principles based on a division of labor—for example, one nurse went through all patients' rooms to check vital signs, two helped all patients prepare for bed, one handed out all medications, and so on. Final responsibility lay with the head nurse, who assigned, coordinated, and controlled the execution of these tasks. The nursing educator, theorist, and nun Liliane Juchli (1933–2020) noted critically in her nursing textbook as early as 1976: "With this system there is a great danger that the patient does not know who is actually responsible for him and his needs. He feels forced into the role of a work object."[26] With the introduction of shift work in the mid-1960 s and functional nursing, psychological symptoms in nurses can be observed for the first

---

[23] Flyer for the demonstration against the hospital regulations on Wednesday, June 9, 1971, collection of photos and press articles from the Children's Hospital at Heidelberg University in the Institute for the History and Ethics of Medicine in Heidelberg. Translation by the author of this article.

[24] "Gesellschaft. Krankenhäuser. Die im Elend," *Der Spiegel* 50, Dec. 7. 1970, 46–62.

[25] "Aus Personalmangel leere Krankenbetten. 'Chirurgie' muß Teile der Station 10 schließen—Schwestern zur Reaktivierung aufgerufen," *Rhein-Neckar-Zeitung*, Sep. 1974.

[26] Liliane Juchli, *Allgemeine und spezielle Krankenpflege. Ein Lehr- und Lernbuch*, 2nd ed. (Stuttgart: Georg Thieme Verlag, 1976), 24–25.

time that resembled today's concept of burnout—for example, nurses showed exhaustion even though they worked significantly fewer hours than in the decades before, as the now fragmented, tightly timed work put more strain on them than providing round-the-clock care for patients with a holistic approach to nursing.[27] Later, functional care was also viewed critically because it happened that nursing measures were forgotten or carried out incorrectly because the division of labor made coordination of the nursing actions complicated.[28]

The Cost-Containment Act of 1977 was intended to further reduce hospital expenditure.[29] This was also associated with savings in personnel costs, so the personnel ratio in nursing was also significantly worsened. The fact that savings potential was seen in nursing staff immediately cancelled out efforts to improve working conditions by recruiting new nursing staff.

In the late 1970 s and early 1980 s, there was an increase in voices in nursing that noted the dehumanization in patient care and called for patient-oriented care.[30] Liliane Juchli propagated the concept of "holistic nursing," which included much more than nursing oriented to the physical and emotional needs of patients. She framed this form of nursing as one that embedded it in "overarching contexts" and rejected old attributions of the self-sacrificing helper. Juchli understood holistic nursing as nursing that is not primarily oriented toward medicine and does not focus on the diagnostic findings, but goes far beyond that. Rather, holistic nursing should be oriented to the individual person, his needs, and his condition, should be on an equal footing with medicine, and should be effective and meaningful, even when medicine can do nothing (more).[31] Juchli, the nursing theorist, thus set herself apart from the fragmented understanding that influenced thinking in biomedicine at the time. She was able to refer to traditions of thought that went back to the 1930 s. The nursing theorist Virginia Henderson (1897–1996), from the United States, already regarded the human being as a whole and based her nursing model on fourteen basic human needs. Juchli transferred Henderson's model to the German-speaking context by intro-

---

[27] Susanne Kreutzer, "Fragmentierung der Pflege. Umbrüche des pflegerischen Handelns in den 1960er Jahren," in *Transformationen pflegerischen Handelns. Institutionelle Kontexte und soziale Praxis vom 19. bis 21. Jahrhundert*, ed. Susanne Kreutzer (Göttingen: V&R Universitätsverlag Osnabrück, 2010), 109–32, at 119–27.

[28] Thomas Elkeles, "Arbeitsorganisation in der Krankenpflege. Zur Kritik an der Funktionspflege," *Kritische Medizin im Argument. Jahrbuch für Kritische Medizin* 13, Special Issue: *Pflege und Krankenhaus. Krankenhaus und Politik. Politik und Gesundheit. Gesundheit und Umfeld* (1988): 5–19.

[29] Wasem, "Zur Entwicklung von Kostendämpfungspolitik und Strukturreformen."

[30] Juchli, *Allgemeine und spezielle Krankenpflege*.

[31] Liliane Juchli, *Ganzheitliche Pflege: Vision oder Wirklichkeit* (Basel, Eberswalde: RECOM-Verlag, 1992), 71.

ducing Henderson's basic needs as "activities of daily living" (ATLs) as fundamental for good nursing in her nursing textbook, which has been published since 1973.[32]

Linked to these demands were those for improving working conditions by increasing nursing staff. Nurses increasingly questioned the ethos of self-sacrificing service to the sick and emphasized that care oriented to the needs of the patient could be provided only if working conditions in nursing were improved.

Conclusion

This chapter has shown the problems that have arisen from a lack of reforms in nursing education and organization, as well as from expansion and austerity policies in the health-care system, the consequences of which we are still noticing today. Demands of the nursing staff have so far received little attention in health policy.

It was not until the COVID-19 pandemic, which made it clear that hospital or intensive care beds could not be used as a resource in the health-care system without sufficient nursing staff, that the importance of well-trained nursing staff was brought into general awareness. In the meantime, the self-image of nurses has finally changed from the concept of loving service to the sick to a professional ethos.

Nurses expressed their professional self-image more strongly in the media during the pandemic than before. Even though the Christian nursing ethos was still present, most nurses emphasized their professionalism and demanded adequate pay and appropriate recognition for their work. Self-sacrificing nursing under pandemic conditions is no longer seen as a desirable ethos, but rather as dangerous for the well-being of patients and their health-care providers. A large number of well-trained nurses will leave the profession if the framework conditions for nursing do not change fundamentally.

---

[32] Liliane Juchli, *Allgemeine und spezielle Krankenpflege. Ein Lehr- und Lernbuch*, 1st ed. (Stuttgart: Georg Thieme Verlag, 1973).

Health-Care Chaplains and Medical Ethics: Clinical and Educational Experiences[1]

Thorsten Moos

Ethics has recently become an increasingly important task in clinical pastoral care. Hospital chaplains are challenged to appropriate ethics as an element of their pastoral professionalism, to develop corresponding skills, and to reflect on their own role in ethical situations and processes in the clinic.

Due to its history, the relationship of pastoral care to ethics is full of tensions. The pastoral-care movement of the twentieth century sought as much as possible to avoid moral judgments in conversations with clients. The pastoral caregiver ought to understand himself or herself no longer as a moral authority, but as a companion on a path to emancipation, whereas morality was often counted among the oppressive forces. However, as pastoral caregivers in the clinic have found themselves increasingly called upon as experts for the normative (sections 1 and 2), ethics again has become a subject of pastoral teaching (section 3). Fundamental problems of clinical ethics—for example, how to deal with the limits of life—raise traditional theological questions in a different manner (section 4). Thus, pastoral caregivers must reconsider the relationship between pastoral care and ethics theologically and develop corresponding professional ethical skills (section 5).

1. A Case Study

A patient is suffering from cancer at a very advanced stage. She is no longer ingesting sufficiently on her own. It has to be decided whether an artificial diet will be given. A simple gastric tube is not possible in this case. Intravenous nutrition could be administered via a portacath, but this is problematic as a per-

---

[1] This chapter was previously published in German as "Seelsorge und Klinische Ethik," in *Handbuch der Krankenhausseelsorge*, ed. Traugott Roser, 5th ed. (Göttingen: Vandenhoeck & Ruprecht, 2019), 334–43, and is included in this volume with kind permission of the publisher.

manent solution. The patient does not explicitly comment on this; moreover, it is not clear to what extent she is really aware of her situation. A conflict arises between her relatives, who demand the portacath, and the treating doctor, who is skeptical and feels pressured and patronized. In this conflict, the doctor involves the hospital chaplain, who for her part does not know the patient.

After talking to the relatives, the chaplain visits the patient at the bedside. In retrospect, she meditates on her visit in an interview:

> If I take a critical look at it again, I would say that I was a bit goal-oriented, which I usually am not in pastoral care. Right, I'm just realizing that. You have to know that this patient ... did not talk of her own accord. Yes, so I had to start somewhere, and I started by asking how she is doing. The breakfast was still on the table, and since it was all about the question of food, I started talking about the visible things, how eating went this morning. And then she said that she takes a bite [of the roll] and then it's enough and then she's fed up. And I was already pursuing the issue of how fed up she is with life as a whole. At which point she sees herself, not directly from what she said about the roll, but that was a road. And if I'm honest now, when I went to see her, I already had in mind that I wanted to have an impression of where the patient actually wants to go.[2]

This quote is revealing in several ways:

1. The focus is on a treatment decision near the end of life. Since the patient does not comment on the situation or is possibly no longer able to comment, other persons come into play: relatives, medical staff, caregivers. A conflict arises among them, which touches on at least two levels: factually, the appropriate treatment, and procedurally, the question of who has to decide about what is appropriate. There is need for communication. An *ethical situation* has popped up.

2. In this case, the attending physician could use the clinical ethics structures and arrange for an ethical case discussion. However, she decides to proceed informally at first. Ethics in the clinic does *not only take place in formal structures of ethics counseling*.

3. The doctor asks the hospital chaplain to come along. Apparently, she trusts her to help solve a moral conflict: She expects *ethical competence* from the pastoral caregiver.

4. The pastor understands this as a mandate, accepts it, and gets in touch with the patient. She tries to determine the patient's will, which is relevant to the

---

[2] The interview was conducted as part of the study "Ethics in Clinic Pastoral Care," the results of which are published in Thorsten Moos et al., *Ethik in der Klinikseelsorge. Empirie, Theologie, Ausbildung* (Göttingen: Vandenhoeck & Ruprecht, 2016); translation by Thorsten Moos. The translation is slightly modified for readability.

issue of further treatment. In this way, she lets her pastoral work be guided by a central medical-ethical and legal category. In the interview, she reflects for the first time that this ethical approach has influenced her acting as a pastoral caregiver. *Pastoral care changes in contact with ethics.*

The implications of this case study will now be developed in detail.

2. The Ethics Boom in the Hospital and Pastoral Care

Ethics in the clinic has experienced a boom in recent decades. The continuously expanded instruments of modern medicine, which open up options for action even in extreme life situations, have led to an increased need for decisions. Much of what used to be "fate" (*Schicksal*) has now become something to actively bring about (*Machsal*, in Odo Marquard's term). At the same time, it has become increasingly clear that patients, relatives, and staff show a plurality of preferences and values. It is not self-evident what is best for this patient in this situation. Conflicts arise in particular where a patient is no longer able to consent to his or her treatment and no relevant written expression of will (patient's provision or medical directive) exists. In this case, the legal figure of the *presumed will* demands high-level interpretations and negotiations from the environment: what would the patient opt for in this situation?

In the past decades, structures of clinical ethics counseling have been successively established, first in the United States and later in Germany. In Germany, the denominational hospitals in particular were important drivers of this development.[3] At the center of clinical ethics counseling there is usually an ethics committee: representatives of different clinical professional groups and hierarchical levels discuss current ethical conflicts *ex ante* or *ex post*, determine general ethical guidelines for processes in the clinic—for example, for dealing with the dying—and organize education on ethical topics. Discussion of current cases of conflict can also take place in consultations on wards, with members of the ethics committee and clinical ethics advisers participating. In all cases, ethics committees have only an advisory function; the final decision about treatment rests with the attending physician. These formal structures of ethics advice have been considerably stabilized and professionalized in recent years: models for the structured course of a case discussion have been developed, advanced training and education have been established, and quality standards have been defined.[4]

---

[3] See also Deutscher Evangelischer Krankenhausverband/Katholischer Krankenhausverband Deutschlands, eds., *Ethik-Komitee im Krankenhaus* (Freiburg, 1997).

[4] See Vorstand der Akademie für Ethik in der Medizin, "Standards für Ethikberatung in Einrichtungen des Gesundheitssystems," *Ethik in der Medizin* 22 (2010): 149–53.

However, there are still significant differences between individual hospitals with regard to the acceptance and actual use of clinical ethics advice.

Typically, case discussions deal with conflicts at the limits of life, that is, with the treatment of patients in the last phase of their lives or of severely ill newborns. Other conflicts arise, for example, in the course of treating people with dementia or with mental illnesses and disorders.

In clinical ethics counseling, hospital chaplains are often involved. They take part in case discussions in various roles: either they have accompanied the patient in question by themselves, and can thus provide an additional professional perspective, or they act as moderators responsible for the entire process or as ethics experts. Clinical ethics counseling is one of the reasons why pastoral caregivers have recently become more intensively involved in the organization of the clinic. Pastoral care no longer operates in a distanced "intermediate space"[5] but is increasingly integrated into the team. This integration is accompanied by an increase in options as well as constraints.[6]

In the clinic, "ethics" is thus primarily understood as an institution firmly anchored in the structures of the organization, providing multiprofessional advice with regard to difficult and potentially conflicting treatment decisions. Interestingly, pastoral caregivers usually have a much broader concept of ethics. When asked about their encounters with "ethics" in the clinic, they name a large spectrum of topics and situations reaching far beyond institutionalized ethics counseling.[7] The above case study shows ethical communication taking place in passing (with the doctor) or at the bedside (with the patient), and in any case beyond any formal counseling session. Situations that pastoral caregivers describe as ethically relevant are not always targeting a specific decision; the issue is often about ethical communication before and after treatment decisions, or about lengthy processes not focused on a single decision. In these situations, explicit deliberation does not always take place; issues are often communicated indirectly. Sometimes an "ethical uneasiness" about the course of treatment emerges, but it remains latent and never explicitly becomes a "case." Moreover, ethics as pastoral caregivers see it is not always about treatment decisions; questions of lifestyle or organizational culture are also considered ethical issues. Finally, rituals such as devotions or fetal burials on the clinic grounds can also function as forums of ethical reflection. This broad concept of ethics is of great importance for the question of a professional relationship between pastoral care and ethics in the clinic.

---

[5] "Zwischen-Raum": see Michael Klessmann, ed., *Handbuch der Krankenhausseelsorge*, 3rd ed. (Göttingen: Vandenhoeck & Ruprecht, 2008), 16.
[6] See Dorothee Haart, *Seelsorge im Wirtschaftsunternehmen Krankenhaus*, Studien zur Theologie und Praxis der Seelsorge 68 (Würzburg: Echter, 2007), 254 ff.
[7] See Moos et al., *Ethik in der Klinikseelsorge*, 52 ff., 268 f.

3. Research Overview

Since the late 1980 s, the topic of ethics has received increasing attention in pastoral care education. This (re-)discovery of ethics is linked to a description of modern society as complex, pluralized, and individualized—a diagnosis that states a need for ethical orientation. It has been realized that ethical questions and conflicts cannot be reduced to psychological constellations but constitute problems of conduct of life with their own logic. In the context of medicine, such questions arise in specific form and intensity. Ethics thus becomes a prominent subject of pastoral care and the subject of pastoral-care education.[8] In the area of clinical pastoral care, even a separate series of books was devoted to its relationship to ethics. Up to now, four volumes have been published which map the field with the help of detailed practical reports, discuss the interfaces between clinical pastoral care and ethics, and analyze the influence of religious pluralism on clinical pastoral care.[9]

While many of these works are programmatic or principle-theoretical in nature, scientific ethics has come to realize in recent decades that the empirical perception of relevant fields is also of great importance for ethics. Therefore, the relationship between clinical pastoral care and ethics has also been investigated in empirical studies. Chaplains are involved in clinical ethics as participants in ethics committees[10] and in a variety of ethical situations in and outside of clinical ethics counseling.[11] Furthermore, the pastoral handling of ethical conflicts was examined as an example for the field of neonatology.[12] The following considerations are due in particular to these empirical insights.

---

[8] See, for example, the special issues of *Pastoraltheologie* 80 (1991) and *Wege zum Menschen* 58 (2006) as well as Ulrich Körtner, *Ethik im Krankenhaus. Diakonie–Seelsorge–Medizin* (Göttingen: Vandenhoeck & Ruprecht, 2007); Traugott Roser et al., eds., *Spiritual Care: Der Beitrag von Seelsorge zum Gesundheitswesen*, 2nd ed. (Stuttgart: Kohlhammer, 2017); and Udo Schlaudraff, "Krankenhausseelsorge und Ethik," in Klessmann, *Handbuch der Krankenhausseelsorge*, 3rd ed., 209–20; also in 4th ed. (2013), 251–62.

[9] Walter Moczynski, Hille Haker, and Katrin Bentele, eds., *Medical Ethics in Health Care Chaplaincy: Essays* (Berlin: Lit, 2009–).

[10] See Reiner Anselm, ed., *Ethik als Kommunikation. Zur Praxis klinischer Ethik-Komitees in theologischer Perspektive* (Göttingen: Universitätsverlag Göttingen, 2008).

[11] See Moos et al., *Ethik in der Klinikseelsorge*.

[12] See Wilfried Sturm, *"Was soll man da in Gottes Namen sagen?" Der seelsorgerliche Umgang mit ethischen Konfliktsituationen im Bereich der Neonatologie und seine Bedeutung für das Verhängnis von Seelsorge und Ethik* (dissertation, Leipzig 2012) (Göttingen: Vandenhoeck & Ruprecht, 2015).

4. Theological Considerations

In the hospital, a large number of ethical questions and problems are touched upon that can be reconstructed theologically. When confronted with these problems, hospital chaplains can bring aspects of the religious rationality of Christianity to the highly professionalized field of clinical ethics. A gesture of theological superiority, however—as if the pastor were the last remaining bastion of independent moral sincerity in an impersonal, mechanized, economized hospital—is not only doomed to fail communicatively but also factually inappropriate. Members of the medical and nursing professions as well as other professional groups in the clinic regularly perceive a gap between their own professional ethical standards and the reality of the organization;[13] and as individuals, employees of the hospital are morally approachable as well. Certainly, what individuals, professions, or medical-ethical texts address as "ethics" is in many respects influenced by Christian ethos and ethical thinking.[14] Nonetheless, clinical ethics is an inescapably secular business in the sense that the validity of principles of medical ethics, professional ethics, or case-related agreements does not depend on theological premises. Both insights are equally decisive for a pastoral hermeneutics of clinical ethics. On one hand, such a hermeneutics can understand many issues and convictions discussed in clinical ethics as *flesh of its own flesh*. On the other hand, it can acknowledge the secular conditions of ethical communication, that is, its aim at general consent. Hospital chaplaincy, then, as a theological enterprise, can contribute for its own sake to the nurturing of a general ethos, to moral sensibility, to an ethical culture of communication, and to pragmatic decision-making.[15] Let us consider three examples.

First, the topic of personality: the unconditional claim of a person to be respected, regardless of his or her empirical constitution, and the ultimate elusiveness and intangibility of a person can be traced back to Christian anthropology. But they can also be found in the spectrum of philosophical concepts of the person and have their counterparts in the medical and nursing ethos. For clinical ethics, the negotiation of personness is of central importance, especially for treatment decisions at the limits of life. It shows that pastoral workers are highly committed at this point.[16]

---

[13] See Roser et al., *Spiritual Care*, 322, 413.

[14] See, for example, Tom L. Beauchamp and James F. Childress, *Principles of Biomedical Ethics*, 7th ed. (New York: Oxford University Press, 2013); and Ulrich Körtner, *Grundkurs Pflegeethik* (Vienna: Facultas, 2004).

[15] For a Christian care of a general ethos, see Ulrich Barth, "Die religiöse Dimension des Ethischen. Grundzüge einer christlichen Verantwortungsethik," in *Religion in der Moderne* (Tübingen: Mohr Siebeck, 2003), 315–44.

[16] See Moos et al., *Ethik in der Klinikseelsorge*, 154 ff., 270 ff.

A second example is the concept of conscience, which is central to theology. This concept has entered medical and nursing professional ethics as well as medical law in a specific manner. The professional independence of the medical profession is addressed as freedom of conscience, and nurses who are in principle bound by instructions may not be obliged against their conscience, for example, to participate in abortions. In common moral semantics, the concept of conscience has largely been replaced by that of responsibility. Nevertheless, in interviews, pastoral caregivers conceive of certain situations in the clinic as being relevant to conscience: namely, when it comes to claiming a space for being a moral subject under difficult conditions.[17] This space can either be internal–for example, when a doctor feels a moral dilemma and expresses it to the pastor–or it can be external–for example, when a nurse feels compelled to act in a certain situation as a moral subject, to openly take a stand and in this way force ethical communication. In questions of conscience, the individual's moral integrity is affected in a way that goes beyond mere moral disagreement. A fundamental question of clinical ethics is to what extent the individual conviction expressed with reference to individual conscience can be communicated to others, and how a complex, differentiated organization optimized for smooth functioning can integrate the strong moral bonds of its members.[18] The theological tradition knows about the ambivalence of conscience between moral fortitude (see the Luther-in-Worms pathos) and fundamentalism. Here, too, hospital chaplains who find themselves addressed in questions of conscience are able to contribute some theologically trained reflexivity.

Third, with the question of individual responsibility in the organization and the increasing need for decision-making in the clinic, the topic of guilt reemerges. It is important to find ways of pastoral care between the criticism of exaggerated and destructive self-attributions of guilt, on one hand, and the acknowledgment of guilt experiences on the other. Anyone who wants to speak theologically of forgiveness must also speak of guilt. The religious exoneration from guilt (*grace*) implicitly presupposes the religious affirmation of guilt (*judgment*): a challenge to pastoral practice.[19]

---

[17] For the following paragraphs, see Moos et al., *Ethik in der Klinikseelsorge*, 129 ff., 273 ff.

[18] See Franz-Josef Bormann and Verena Wetzstein, eds., *Gewissen. Dimensionen eines Grundbegriffs medizinischer Ethik* (Berlin: De Gruyter, 2014).

[19] See Thorsten Moos, "Eine verlorene Kategorie? Zum Umgang mit moralischer Schuld in der Klinikseelsorge," *Praktische Theologie* 51 (2016): 214–20; and Renja Rentz et al., *Schuld in der Seelsorge. Historische Perspektiven und gegenwärtige Praxis* (Stuttgart: Kohlhammer, 2016).

5. Ethical Competence in Pastoral Care

When dealing with ethics in the clinic, pastoral care needs ethical competence: there is a broad consensus on this.[20] Ethical competence must be successively developed in pastoral training, further training, and continuing education.[21] Literature usually lists ethical competence alongside other pastoral competences, such as theological, communicative, and pastoral-psychological competence.[22] Such assignment implies that ethics is an additional element of pastoral professionalism, standing outside the core area of pastoral care that is conceived of as a theologically and psychologically trained art of conversation. This concept is supported by the fact that ethics in the clinic does in fact require a broad range of field-specific knowledge and skills. These include fluency in dealing with clinical processes, legal requirements (medical indication, patient rights, presumed will, etc.), as well as ethical and medical-ethical instruments (such as models of ethical advice and their ethical foundations).[23] In order to develop ethical competencies in this sense, specific education and training modules are offered for hospital chaplains or for medical professionals in general.[24]

However, the introductory case study shows that ethical competence in clinical pastoral care encompasses more than a set of *additional* knowledge and skills. First, it is noticeable that the pastoral caregiver is open to overtones when talking to the patient about food intake: how fed up is the patient with life? So she uses a central pastoral competence, the hermeneutics of metaphorical speech, in an ethical context. Along this line, it can be shown empirically that pastoral caregivers use a variety of classical pastoral skills—of communication,

---

[20] However, there are important general objections to a strong focus on competence in pastoral care, which is thought to overemphasize professional expertise and thus to neglect the personal aspect of pastoral care. See Dorothee Lange, "Evangelische Seelsorge in ethischen Konfliktsituationen," *Pastoraltheologie* 80 (1991): 62–77, here at 77; and Dietrich Rössler, *Grundriss der praktischen Theologie*, 2nd ed. (Berlin: De Gruyter, 1994), 202–06.

[21] Ulrich Körtner developed a multistage model of ethical competence. See Körtner, *Ethik im Krankenhaus*.

[22] See Traugott Roser, "Ethik in der Klinikseelsorge. Neue Herausforderungen der Seelsorgelehre," in *Grenzen überschreiten*, ed. Trutz Rendtorff, Roger Busch, and Nikolaus Knoepffler (Munich: Utz, 2001), 77–89, at 87 f.; and Hartmut Wortmann, Thomas Jarck, and Ulrike Mummenhoff, eds., *Qualitätshandbuch zur Krankenhausseelsorge* (Göttingen: Vandenhoeck & Ruprecht, 2010), 48 ff.

[23] See Andrea Dörries et al., eds., *Klinische Ethikberatung. Ein Praxisbuch für Krankenhäuser und Einrichtungen der Altenpflege*, 2nd ed. (Stuttgart: Kohlhammer, 2010).

[24] See, for example, the activities of the Center for Health Ethics (Zentrum für Gesundheitsethik), Hannover.

theological interpretation, and liturgical action—when they are confronted with ethical questions. Equipped with their "old" pastoral tools, hospital chaplains enter an ethical space and experience new demands to cope with the tensions and fault lines of this space. As shown, theological categories such as *the person* or *the conscience* have ethical implications that need to be reflected upon. The same applies to liturgical acts: how is guilt articulated, for example, when a fetus is buried?[25] Pastoral care takes place under the tension between moral reluctance, on one hand, and moral positioning on the other hand. Another tension emerges between the articulation of ambiguity, on one hand, and the production of unambiguity due to the situational requirements—a decision has to be made!—on the other. All of this must be taken into professional consideration. It is therefore important not only to acquire additional ethical skills but also to further develop established pastoral skills *as* ethical skills.[26]

But the case study also shows something else: the pastoral caregiver realizes in the interview situation that her work has changed. She comes to the bedside with an attitude that is no longer merely client-centered. Rather, she works with an external mandate: she wants to find out what the patient *wants* with regard to her continued life and her further treatment. In doing so, she is pursuing a morally valuable goal: she wants to give the patient a voice in the conflict between doctors and relatives. Nevertheless, serious questions can be asked about her role as a pastoral caregiver: should she have accepted this mandate? Should she have interpreted it like that? Should she have communicated it to the patient? Under what conditions can such a doubly commissioned conversation succeed?

These questions address a third element of ethical competence in clinical pastoral care: caregivers need the ability to reflect on the development of their own ethical role. What at first glance appears as a tension between pastoral care and ethics reveals itself on closer inspection as a tension between different pastoral care roles—and at the same time as a tension between different approaches to ethics. The ethical *metacompetence* required here affects the allocation of ethics and pastoral care as well as the moral involvement of pastoral caregivers in ethical conflicts or their position in multiprofessional ethical communication.[27] The training of ethical competence in this sense, as well as the previously mentioned development of pastoral competences *as* ethical competences, proves necessary not only in hospital chaplaincy but also in other fields of pastoral care. Its education should therefore be included in basic pastoral care training.[28]

---

[25] See Roser, *Spiritual Care*, 224–32.
[26] Moos et al., *Ethik in der Klinikseelsorge*, 304–08.
[27] Ibid., 308–11.
[28] For this purpose, the "Heidelberg Module" for the training of ethical competence was developed and tested; see Moos et al., *Ethik in der Klinikseelsorge*, 313 ff.

6. Final Remark

Clinical ethics as a field of pastoral care is likely to gain even more importance in the future. At the same time, with the institutionalization (and financing) of clinical ethics, other professional groups show themselves responsible for ethical issues in the hospital. Academically trained medical ethicists, practical philosophers, and physicians also claim their professional competence in, if not ownership of, clinical ethics. At the same time, the academic consolidation of medical ethics through degree programs, publications, and professional societies is associated with a narrowing of ethics towards a decision-making technique in difficult treatments. At the beginning of its popularity in the hospital, the term "ethics" served as a legitimation for communication about problems in the hospital in a very broad sense. In the meantime, its legitimizing function has generally become much narrower. In contrast, the broad concept of ethics that pastoral caregivers bring to the clinic due to their job-specific range of roles is an important corrective. This corresponds to the fact that pastoral caregivers in the clinic themselves act as personal legitimators of communication—as a kind of personal ethics committee in passing. *You are allowed to talk to hospital chaplains.* This is one of the reasons why clinical pastoral care is a high ethical good in itself.

Medical Anthropology and Theology on Human Destiny

Gregor Etzelmüller

The Heidelberg physician and philosopher Viktor von Weizsäcker (1886-1957)[1] pointed out a paradox: from a scientific perspective, patients may be fully healed, yet they often resist considering themselves healthy—and they are not wrong. They

> "do not admit that they are healthy now, and they are quite right. For the knowledge of how a sickness came to be does not provide them personally with a new sense of direction. So they rightly ask, what am I supposed to do now in order to become truly healthy?"[2]

In asking this way, people show that health is not a neutral state in relation to the many paths a person may take in life; for every person, to be healthy means to follow some particular course in life. Fundamentally these people ask for the destiny of their lives. In doing so, they challenge physicians to expand the boundaries of their professional expertise. For Weizsäcker, at this point medi-

---

[1] Viktor von Weizsäcker was, after periods of assistance with Johannes Adolf von Kries in Freiburg and Ludolf von Krehl in Heidelberg, from 1920 until 1941 head of the neurological department at the Medical Clinic in Heidelberg, from 1941 to 1945 full professor of neurology and head of the Otfried Foerster Institute in Breslau, and from then until his retirement in 1952 professor of general clinical medicine in Heidelberg. He is the founder of anthropological medicine in Germany. The theory of this form of psychosomatic medicine is medical anthropology. As a first introduction, see Hartwig Wiedebach, "Some Aspects of a Medical Anthropology, Pathic Existence and Causality in Viktor von Weizsäcker," *Historical Psychiatry* 20 (2009): 360-76; Udo Benzenhöfer, *Der Arztphilosoph Viktor von Weizsäcker. Leben und Werk im Überblick* (Göttingen: Vandenhoeck & Ruprecht, 2007).

[2] Viktor von Weizsäcker, "Fälle und Probleme: Anthropologische Vorlesungen in der Medizinischen Klinik," in *Fälle und Probleme: Klinische Vorstellungen*, Gesammelte Schriften 9 (Frankfurt: Suhrkamp, 1988), 8-276, 222.

cine borders on theology. Medicine continues to require dialogue with theology. "We approach theology in order to ask questions, in order to receive instruction about the meaning of the ultimate human destiny."[3] What the physician Weizsäcker had in mind here was nothing less than "what the Apostle [Paul] called the resurrection of the body."[4]

Hoping to find out about human destiny, Weizsäcker did not seek dialogue with theology merely for personal reasons, although he was a Christian from a Christian-shaped family.[5] Rather, his choice of a partner in dialogue makes sense also from a historical and systematic perspective. Historically, the modern discourse about human destiny has its origins in the treatise *Considerations about the Destiny of the Human Person* (*Betrachtung über die Bestimmung des Menschen*, 1748) by the German Enlightenment theologian Johann Joachim Spalding (1714–1804).[6] Within less than fifty years, the tractate was printed in eleven editions. "The title of this treatise, which was published again and again, provided the German Enlightenment with the cue for one of its most characteristic basic ideas."[7]

Spalding's treatise further shows why theology is the relevant discipline in which to discuss the topic of human destiny. Spalding points out that it is not a foregone conclusion that people who do what their destiny requires[8] will in fact reach their destiny. Should death have the last word, the righteous soul would be "forever robbed of the natural happy consequences of its inner rectitude." Too often virtue finds its reward "in pain and torture, at the hands of cruel hangmen

---

[3] Weizsäcker, "Von den seelischen Ursachen der Krankheit," in *Körpergeschehen und Neurose: Psychosomatische Medizin*, Gesammelte Schriften 6 (Frankfurt: Suhrkamp, 1986), 399–417, 406.

[4] Ibid., 401.

[5] See Peter Achilles, "Konvergenzen zwischen Medizin und Theologie: Zu Biographie und Werk Viktor von Weizsäckers," in *Die Wahrheit der Begegnung: Anthropologische Perspektiven der Neurologie. Festschrift Dieter Janz*, ed. Rainer-M. E. Jacobi (Würzburg: Königshausen & Neumann, 2001), 250–66.

[6] Johann Joachim Spalding, *Betrachtung über die Bestimmung des Menschen*, in *Die Bestimmung des Menschen*, ed. Albrecht Beutel et al. (Tübingen: Mohr Siebeck, 2006), 1–25.

[7] Clemens Schwaiger, "Zur Frage nach den Quellen von Spaldings 'Bestimmung des Menschen': Ein ungelöstes Rätsel der Aufklärungsforschung," *Aufklärung* 11, no. 1 (1999): 7–19, 7.

[8] For Spalding, humans need to direct all their efforts toward the "happiness of the human species" (*Betrachtung über die Bestimmung des Menschen*, 11 f.). There is a "legislator in me" who demands "justice toward all people, rectitude in my entire conduct, gratitude toward my native country and benefactors, generosity even toward enemies, and a general love in the widest sense of the term" (ibid., 12). This and subsequent translations are mine (G.E.).

acting at the command of even more cruel tyrants."[9] "There is a kind of disharmony here," Spalding judges, "which undoubtedly would be a mistake if it were not to dissolve in complete peace later on."[10] The question of human destiny requires the perspective of eternal life, which would fulfill the human destiny, "which is to be righteous, and to flourish within this righteousness."[11] The question for human destiny is not exhausted in the question of how I should act, but it implies another one—of what I can hope for. For that reason, it is part of religion and must be discussed in theology.

Since the discipline of medicine knows that in life we are first affected before we actively intervene in the world, Weizsäcker sees a close affinity between medicine and theology. In both fields, people know that our action cannot secure the attainment of our human destiny. We continue to depend on external help.

Further, it is crucial for Weizsäcker that such help reaches the real person, that is, bodily, embodied humans. Precisely as a physician, he understands that according to Paul, human destiny is nothing less than bodily resurrection.[12] He argued that "death and the resurrection of the body are clearly opposed to the inordinate spiritualism of the church, and neither must we forget that Jesus steps forward as a savior and physician of bodily ailments." Since both medicine and theology place "the mystery of embodiment" at the center, Weizsäcker considered "the medical faculty, not the philosophical one, most closely related to the theological faculty."[13]

1. Human Destiny in the Light of Pauline Theology

Paul does in fact envision human destiny as an existence characterized by abiding embodiment. For him, the person is destined to be shaped by God's Spirit, communicating faith, hope, and love in bodily actions. The human destiny lies in becoming a spiritual body (*sōma pneumatikon*; 1 Cor. 15:44).

---

[9] Ibid., 19.
[10] Ibid., 20.
[11] Ibid., 25.
[12] A resurrection of the body was unthinkable for Spalding: "These limbs that constitute my organs, they are not *myself*; according to my clear sensation, they are distinct from *myself*. My true self is that in myself which has impressions, makes judgments, resolves to do things" (ibid., 21). For that reason, Spalding suggests, the true person will not be lost in physical death (ibid., 22).
[13] Viktor von Weizsäcker, "Begegnungen und Entscheidungen," in *Natur und Geist: Begegnungen und Entscheidungen*, Gesammelte Schriften 1 (Frankfurt: Suhrkamp, 1986), 191–399, 306.

Paul views the bodies of believers as temples of the Holy Spirit (1 Cor. 6:19). As the congregation is one body that constitutes God's temple in 1 Corinthians 3:16, so it is every individual body in 1 Corinthians 6 that is the dwelling place of the Holy Spirit. The temple in Jerusalem was understood as God's "dwelling place," which was "the source of life-giving water, which safeguards the persistence of nature and society."[14] According to the Old Testament scholar Erich Zenger, the manifold semantic images of temple theology at bottom present variations on one central theme: "The temple, the place of God's presence, is the privileged source of life and salvation. Those who are in the area of the temple itself or in its proximity literally participate in the divine power of life."[15]

When Paul explicitly calls the body of the believer a temple, he goes back to this idea: believers not only participate in the divine power of life; their bodies as temples of the Holy Spirit will even become sources of life and flourishing themselves. All around them, nature and people will thrive.

This also goes to show that Paul's image of the body as a temple does not describe some given essence of the human person, but it aims at what God calls humans to become. The "body of sin" (Rom. 6:6) is destined to become the temple of the Holy Spirit. God intends for humans to transcend their evolutionary advanced socialization so that they communicate faith, hope, and love instead.

In Paul's talk of Christians as the temple of God or the temple of the Holy Spirit, the Apostle sometimes focuses on the congregation as one body and sometimes on the individual body of the believer. This shows how individual believers and the congregation mutually depend on each other. Without individual believers, no congregation could develop—but without the congregation, nobody would come to believe in Christ either. In order to become a temple of the Holy Spirit, a person depends on an environment that promotes life and enables such growth. The Christian congregation wants to win people over for its vision, or more precisely, for the good aspirations that God has for creation. However, as individual believers contribute to the edification of the congregation as well, we see that the point of salvation does not consist in the deliverance of individuals, but in the building up of a community characterized by faith, hope, and love.[16] In

---

[14] Beate Ego, "Der Strom der Tora: Zur Rezeption eines tempeltheologischen Motivs in frühjüdischer Zeit," in *Gemeinde ohne Tempel—Community without Temple: Zur Substituierung und Transformation des Jerusalemer Tempels und seines Kultes im Alten Testament, antiken Judentum und frühen Christentum*, Wissenschaftliche Untersuchungen zum Neuen Testament, ed. Beate Ego (Tübingen: Mohr Siebeck, 1999), 205–14, 209.

[15] Erich Zenger, "Wer wird Segen empfangen? Psalm 24: Übersetzung und Auslegung," *Bibel und Kirche* 58 (2003): 71–80, 72.

[16] This should be emphasized in contrast to certain trends within Protestantism that understand faith in a radically individualistic sense, tending to lose from view the church as the communion of saints. See Ola Sigurdson, *Heavenly Bodies: Incarnation, the Gaze,*

this sense, the purpose of individuals is to contribute to the building up and the preservation of such a community by becoming such sources of faith, hope, and love themselves, in their individual bodily lives.

For Paul, the triad of faith, hope, and love suggests "a new *Gestalt* of authentic life lived in wholeness according to God's will."[17] In the opening section of what many scholars consider his first letter, Paul thanks God for the faith, love, and hope of the Christians in Thessalonica (1 Thess. 1:3; similarly, Col. 1:4f., Eph. 1:15,18). Similarly, at the end of the letter, he encourages the congregation to continue to abide in faith, love, and hope (1 Thess. 5:8, see also Heb. 6:10–12, 10:22–24). In 1 Corinthians, Paul uses the terms faith, hope, and love again to describe the reality in the congregation that has been given by the Spirit and which will remain in eternity. We also find this triad in Romans (Rom. 5:1–3). According to Paul, human persons are meant to live a life filled with faith, hope, and love—leading to a life that also communicates faith, hope, and love.

In this sense, we can then say that human persons are destined to communicate faith, hope, and love and to build congregations and communities shaped by these attitudes—and to contribute to the building up and preservation of social systems in which justice, mercy, and the knowledge of God—or in a secular idiom, the search for truth—are vital factors.[18]

2. The Wisdom of the Lived Body

After we have seen what medicine can learn from theology according to the quest of human destiny, I want now to show what theology can learn from medicine. A medical anthropology can open up our eyes to the wisdom of our real lived body.

In 1946, Viktor von Weizsäcker wrote:

---

and *Embodiment in Christian Theology* (Grand Rapids: Eerdmans, 2016), 391–5: "The Disappearing Church."

[17] Thomas Söding, *Die Trias Glaube, Hoffnung, Liebe bei Paulus: Eine exegetische Studie*, Stuttgarter Bibelstudien (Stuttgart: Katholisches Bibelwerk, 1992), 163; see Sigrid Brandt, "Sünde: Ein Definitionsversuch," in *Sünde: Ein unverständlich gewordenes Thema*, ed. Sigrid Brandt et al. (Neukirchen: Neukirchener, 1997), 13–34, 20f.

[18] This perspective is fruitful also in a secular discourse; after all, in the face of the current political crises, Martha C. Nussbaum, a thinker within political liberalism, "suggests strategies for nourishing hope, faith, and love of humanity, just when it seems especially difficult to believe that these good emotions might possibly guide us." Nussbaum, *The Monarchy of Fear: A Philosopher Looks at Our Political Crisis* (New York: Simon & Schuster, 2018), 15.

> If I now survey the medical aspect in that period of life that is mine, from 1906 to 1946, the overwhelming power of the bodily human situation is what I find most impressive. It is the dependence of the mind on the body, of the soul on instinct; yet it's also the sagacity of this bodily condition ... wisdom working within matter; how nature comes to the aid of the spirit. ... It's this view on humanity that thwarts the separation of nature and spirit.[19]

The body is not merely an object to which I relate, but as my lived body, it guides me through my world. It opens up my world for me,[20] it opens me up toward others, lets me sense an atmosphere immediately, and often reacts appropriately through intuition—it also enlivens my mind.[21] One of the current leading thinkers on embodiment, Shaun Gallagher, emphasizes that

> "the normal and healthy subject can in large measure forget about her body in the normal routine of the day. The body takes care of itself, and in doing so, it enables the subject to attend, with relative ease, to other practical aspects of life. To the extent that the body effaces itself, it grants to the subject a freedom to think of other things."[22]

Our lived bodies relieve us of the burden of having to control all the steps of our lives consciously. Thus, they give us the freedom to invest our conscious attention in more complex matters and relations beyond everyday routines. My corporeal lived body keeps me alive, enables me to act intentionally, opens up my

---

[19] Viktor von Weizsäcker, "Die Medizin im Streit der Fakultäten," in Weizsäcker, *Grundfragen medizinischer Anthropologie: Allgemeine Medizin*, Gesammelte Schriften 7 (Frankfurt: Suhrkamp, 1987), 197–211, 202.

[20] See James R. Mensch, *Embodiments: From the Body to the Body Politic* (Evanston: Northwestern University Press, 2009), 42, who speaks of our bodily capabilities, "the bodily 'I can'": "Thus, the fact that I have eyes means that I can see some object. That I have legs means that I can move closer to get a better look; that I have hands with fingers allows me to pick it up and manipulate it if it is not too heavy. The same holds for all of our other bodily activities. They give us our access to the world."

[21] This is a common experience of many people in countless life situations. This is not to deny that there are also other experiences in which the body becomes a burden and, as a pain-ridden body, makes life almost impossible. The knowledge of such real experiences should help one perceive the dependence on one's own body, where it can be felt as a gift, with greater gratitude—and to realize one's own bodily dependence in such a way that those who suffer from their bodies receive all humanly possible help. Where pain destroys language, others have to verbalize this pain as a critique of reality.

[22] Shaun Gallagher, *How the Body Shapes the Mind*, 2nd ed. (Oxford: Oxford University Press, 2013), 55.

world to me in immediate ways, and funds my intelligence in acting and perceiving in advance of my conscious efforts.

The wisdom of the lived body is on display, last but not least, when psychosomatic medicine explores how the lived body can contribute to the solution of conflicts. We can observe the wisdom of the lived body even in disease.

According to Weizsäcker, who is de facto among the founders of psychosomatic medicine—even while maintaining a reservation against the term itself—the ill person encounters the physician as a psychosomatic unity. The patient faces the physician as an object, but since it is the patient who asks the physician for help, a subject emerges within the object.[23] The physician can only do justice to this phenomenon, the ill person in her psychosomatic unity, with a therapy that does not separate the disease from the ill person. Rather, the disease needs to be understood in the entirety of the person's life. For that reason, the physician needs to know in equal measure about the anatomic, physiological, psychic, and social factors contributing to the disease, even if their interplay remains unknown.[24] We have "to see a story in every ill person, in the course of which each of two things enters to define the condition: a psychogenesis of bodily phenomena and a somatogenesis of psychic phenomena."[25] For this reason, it is necessary to explore the genesis of a condition in order to understand it. To do so, a circular movement is required, from the area of psychology to the one of physics and chemistry and vice versa.[26]

For such a method, Weizsäcker coined the term *psychobiographic.*[27] It is the specific characteristic of this method to understand "the meaning of the illness" in grasping the physical and the psychic aspects of the illness "in their unity."[28] If both the psychic and the physical aspects together constitute the condition, its characteristics come into view precisely neither through the scientific perspective alone nor through the explicit comments of the patient alone. The physician should focus neither solely on the *Körper*, the body in the third-person perspective of scientific medicine, nor solely on the *Leib*, the body image of the patient, but on the *Leibkörper*, the body schema, the lived body, which is related to my

---

[23] See Viktor von Weizsäcker, *Der kranke Mensch: Eine Einführung in die Medizinische Anthropologie*, in *Fälle und Probleme: Klinische Vorstellungen*, Gesammelte Schriften 9 (Frankfurt: Suhrkamp, 1988), 311–641, 515.
[24] See Weizsäcker, "Krankengeschichte," in *Der Arzt und der Kranke: Stücke einer medizinischen Anthropologie*, Gesammelte Schriften 5 (Frankfurt: Suhrkamp, 1987), 48–66, 52; see Weizsäcker, "Die Schmerzen," in *Der Arzt und der Kranke*, 27–47, 46.
[25] Weizsäcker, *Der kranke Mensch*, 311–641, 504.
[26] See "Die Grundlagen der Medizin," in Weizsäcker, *Grundfragen medizinischer Anthropologie*, 7–28, 24.
[27] Weizsäcker, *Der kranke Mensch*, 629.
[28] Ibid.

own intentions. The *Leibkörper*, the body schema, in this sense—my body and its organs—have a say in the search for the meaning of the illness. "So if someone has gastric ulcers, we try to read off from the physical process what has been the matter also with this person's psychic life."[29] Illness can then be experienced in such a way that potentially, "a psychic development is set in motion through a bodily event."[30] In an illness, truth can come to light.[31]

For precisely that reason, Weizsäcker advocates for a change in attitude toward illness in medicine.

> The old attitude of "let's get rid of this" needs to be replaced by the mindset that says, "yes, but not in this way." Saying "yes" to what the body is trying to communicate, yet making the caveat, "but not in this way," regarding the way the body communicates its message, that is, regarding the way the body has the illness stand in for what it wants to say.[32]

The old attitude toward disease that aims at the elimination of a defect could end up squandering the learning opportunity that the disease presents precisely in the form of a crisis.

For Weizsäcker, it is thus crucial to recognize the competence and the power of the lived body even in the course of a disease. For the transformation of a psychic conflict into a physical disease can contribute to the recovery of the whole person. "Unconsciously," the person "flees from an intolerable situation into an illness," replacing "the psychic conflict with a physical surrender ... and the body renders the service—of going on living, recovering, and beginning anew."[33] Physicians describe similar processes today as well:

> "The serious accident, the intensive care unit, the long stay in the hospital, the sudden change of the previous social structure that is beyond our influence—these factors make possible a kind of catharsis, occasionally leading to a complex reorganization of life."[34]

---

[29] Ibid.
[30] Weizsäcker, "Krankengeschichte," 65; see Weizsäcker, "Die Medizin im Streit der Fakultäten," in Weizsäcker, *Grundfragen medizinischer Anthropologie*, 197–211, 202.
[31] See Weizsäcker, "Über medizinische Anthropologie," in *Der Arzt und der Kranke*, 177–94, 179; and Weizsäcker, *Der kranke Mensch*, 511, 565.
[32] Weizsäcker, "Das Problem des Menschen in der Medizin," in *Grundfragen medizinischer Anthropologie*, 366–71, 369f.; and Weizsäcker, *Der kranke Mensch*, 318f.
[33] Weizsäcker, "Von den seelischen Ursachen der Krankheit," in *Körpergeschehen und Neurose: Psychosomatische Medizin*, Gesammelte Schriften 6 (Frankfurt: Suhrkamp, 1986), 399–417, 409; and Weizsäcker, *Der kranke Mensch*, 500.
[34] Bernd Hontschik, *Körper, Seele, Mensch: Versuch über die Kunst des Heilens* (Frankfurt: Suhrkamp, 2006), 64; see also 49–67.

In expressing psychic conflicts in its own behavior, the lived body can initiate conscious psychic developments through a disease. For Weizsäcker, a disease can alert a person to the fact that she is leading a false life. The medical condition can be experienced as "an offering of knowledge of the truth."[35] Weizsäcker describes two processes: the body's escape into an organic disease that stands in for the solution of a psychosocial conflict, with an ensuing bodily therapy, as well as the view of illness disclosing truth. Both aspects of illness illustrate the enormous capabilities of the lived body in assisting in solving psychic and social conflicts. Nevertheless, the lived body's strategy is highly risky: fleeing into illness, the body brings a form of death into the arena to which it may in fact succumb. For it is not a foregone conclusion that the lived body can stage a genuine illness while avoiding death. Accordingly, Weizsäcker himself pointed out that the meaning of an illness can also lie in disclosing "repressed tendencies to self-harm and self-annihilation."[36] The flight into illness can then be understood in analogy to suicide: the lived body flees into illness, though not in order to recover but to die. Here the lived body does not aid the melancholic soul, but lends expression to it in such a way that results in death.

What the lived body wants to say through its expressive behavior—that is, in the illness—is what Weizsäcker called the meaning of the illness. Unlike classical modern medicine, which focuses on illness as a meaningless phenomenon, anthropological medicine asks what illness wants to bring to light. Weizsäcker wanted to guide (future) physicians to always act as if "every illness has a meaning."[37]

---

[35] Weizsäcker, "Krankengeschichte," 65.
[36] Weizsäcker, *Der kranke Mensch*, 615.
[37] Ibid., 319. Note that the sentence is formulated in the subjunctive in German: "Jede Krankheit habe einen Sinn." It is not a dogmatic statement, but rather a heuristic instruction. In my opinion, this view must be complemented with the conviction that not every illness offers insight into a deeper meaning. There are meaningless illnesses. See Gregor Etzelmüller, "Der kranke Mensch als Thema theologischer Anthropologie: Die Herausforderung der Theologie durch die anthropologische Medizin Viktor von Weizsäckers," *Zeitschrift für Evangelische Ethik* 53 (2009): 163-76, 172-4, 174: "We happen upon the potential meaninglessness of an illness when we see that the lived body, by manifesting a death-wish, becomes an agent of death, when we see that, under the power of sin, the lived body often cannot do anything but point out that this world is falling short of its destiny—and the ill person derives no benefit from this insight. Weizsäcker himself has pointed out that the meaning of an illness often remains opaque (Der kranke Mensch, pp. 548. 579. 595. 602). However, his conviction that there is nothing in the organic world that lacks meaning (Weizsäcker, "Ich und Umwelt in der Erkrankung," in *Der Arzt und der Kranke*, 310-17, 314), did not permit him to deduce the fact of meaningless from the hiddenness of meaning." However, modern classical medicine

To avoid misunderstandings, it is necessary to explain this sentence: That every illness has a meaning means that the lived body always makes a meaningful statement. However, the disease does not have "meaning" insofar as it causes suffering. Illness does not make sense in itself. Illnesses are evils, but the evils that become visible in illnesses are by no means limited to the diseases that conventional medicine diagnoses; rather, the further circumstances of life are also an evil, although we do not perceive them as such. The illness is meaningful in its instrumental use, insofar as it brings to light what has been going on in a person's life and environment, that this person has become ill.

The (possible) meaning of an illness is grasped in the relationship between physician and patient. In order to understand the meaning, a physician must be consulted. For in order to hear what the body is trying to say with the illness, it is necessary to understand the dialects that the organs speak—that is, to recognize how specific organs and their symptoms refer to specific, larger psychic problems. The point is not simply to understand the physical side in the light of the psychic side, but similarly to understand the psychic side in the light of the physical side. Yet the meaning of an illness "can only be realized from the patient's perspective; the physician must not dictate the meaning. For the ill person, the meaning can only be salutary; for the physician, it can only be a plight."[38] The meaning can only be grasped in dialogue with the ill person, and the meaning has only been grasped rightly if the understanding in fact contributes to healing. For precisely this reason, it is part of the physician's task to expose misleading assumptions when the patient and her environment ascribe a meaning to a disease that does not help understand the disease and contribute to a cure. In this way, Weizsäcker critiques rightly "cruelties in moral theology like the belief that diseases are sent by God so that someone may believe in God."[39]

In recent years, there has been an increasing tendency in psychotherapy to draw on the wisdom of the lived body. At the base of this effort has been the insight not only that a person's mood shapes physical expressions, but that a change in physical expressions and posture also influences a person's emotions. Paul Ekman pointed out the phenomenon of facial feedback, for example. "Feedback via the facial muscles," he explains, "causes changes in the brain that caus-

---

assumes the possible meaninglessness all too unreflectively, therefore often treating symptoms instead of causes and thus contributing to the development of chronic diseases. It is important to ask about the possible meaning of the illness, especially at the beginning of a patient's story.

[38] Weizsäcker, "Krankengeschichte," 66.

[39] Ibid.; see also Weizsäcker, "Grundfragen medizinischer Anthropologie," in *Grundfragen medizinischer Anthropologie*, 255–82, 273f.

es emotions in keeping with the current facial expression."⁴⁰ By consciously trying to smile in melancholy moments, one can experience this effect relatively easily. Researchers have demonstrated that a change in the facial muscles shows an effect even when the expression was not changed with the intention to lighten up one's mood.⁴¹ Meanwhile, there has been experimental evidence that emotions can be triggered or prevented not only with a change in facial expressions but also in body posture—a phenomenon called body feedback. This knowledge has been used for therapeutic purposes, but also in acting classes.⁴²

These insights have caused rethinking among psychotherapists.⁴³ Rather than focusing mainly on cognitive processes, they increasingly turn their attention to the body. Those who disregard the body accept at least that ongoing body feedback processes continually undermine the goals they are striving for with cognitive methods. On the other hand, by using bodily exercises in a targeted way, practitioners can reduce stress in patients, evoke particular emotions, and thus support—or even enable—certain cognitive processes.

Further, it would be a significant advance not only to realize the power of the body and to attempt to use it in an instrumental sense, but also to give the corporeal lived body its own say in therapy. When people become attentive to their corporeal lived bodies, they become aware of how they are truly feeling. Mediated by their lived bodies, they come into contact with their innermost desires and sentiments—and in therapy, some do so for the first time in their lives.⁴⁴ Giving people access to themselves, people's lived bodies give them "security and identity" and put them "in touch with reality and with possibilities of control." Patients who have felt like nothing but "puppet[s] controlled by others" thus recover a sense of authorship in their own lives, "in bodily perception and the action resulting from that."⁴⁵ Perception of one's lived body unlocks a per-

---

⁴⁰ Maja Storch, "Wie Embodiment in der Psychologie erforscht wurde," in *Embodiment: Die Wechselwirkung von Körper und Psyche verstehen und nutzen*, ed. Maja Storch et al., 2nd ed. (Bern: Hogrefe, 2010), 35–72, 40.

⁴¹ See Fritz Strack et al., "Inhibiting and Facilitating Conditions of the Human Smile: A Nonobtrusive Test of the Facial Feedback Hypothesis," *Journal of Personality and Social Psychology* 54 (1988): 768–77.

⁴² See Storch, "Wie Embodiment in der Psychologie erforscht wurde," 44–49.

⁴³ See Wolfgang Tschacher and Maja Storch, "Embodiment und Körperpsychotherapie," in *Körperzentrierte Psychotherapie im Dialog: Grundlagen, Anwendungen, Integration. Der IKP-Ansatz von Yvonne Maurer*, ed. Alfred Künzler et al. (Heidelberg: Springer, 2010), 161–75, 161f.

⁴⁴ See Claudia Böttcher, "Burnout," in Künzler et al., *Körperzentrierte Psychotherapie im Dialog*, 193–204, 201.

⁴⁵ Ibid.

son's own resources in problem solving, and the role of the therapist changes as she helps "discover and develop" these resources.[46]

We must not lose from view, of course, that the perception of one's own lived body is once again embodied, which means that it depends on capabilities that can be so restricted that people may not even be able to feel their own lived bodies anymore.

> If there are initial interfering factors already at this stage, such as symptoms of a depression or heavy substance abuse, then these symptoms must be treated first, in some circumstances with pharmaceuticals like antidepressants or anxiolytics, which have a calming effect. This goes to show that the treatment of burnout must be handled by medically qualified experts, that is, psychotherapists with a background as physicians, or by psychologists who work closely with physicians.[47]

In the aftermath of therapy, people are confronted with the task of recovering trust in the lived body, understanding its apparent lack of functioning not as an obstacle, but seeing relevant bodily signals as "warning lights."[48]

There is a significant relationship between this understanding of the lived body and Paul's theology. When discussing social grievances in the celebration of Communion in 1 Corinthians, Paul also remarks on a higher incidence of disease and death in the congregation in Corinth (1 Cor. 11:30 f.). Here Paul's point is that the Corinthians should not simply have tolerated the increasing number of diseases and deaths; rather, they should have taken these as an occasion to ask what it was that made people ill in the first place.

3. The Lived Body as a Critic of the Congregation

The psychosomatic insight into the wisdom of the lived body, even in the form of an illness, is not unknown to Paul. Since Paul describes the human person as a *sōma psychikon*, as a psychosomatic unity (see 1 Cor. 15:44), it is no coincidence that we encounter this insight in his work. According to Paul, the wisdom of the lived body not only consists in the fact that its critique is directed against particular aspects of one's individual life, but also against certain developments in communal life. In 1 Corinthians, Paul comments on an increased incidence of illness in the congregation, and he attributes this fact to abuses in the congre-

---

[46] Tschacher and Storch, "Embodiment und Körperpsychotherapie," 169.
[47] Böttcher, "Burnout," 202.
[48] Ibid., 201.

gation's practice of celebrating Communion (see 1 Cor. 11:28–30).[49] He interprets this crisis as a consequence of a psychosocial conflict. In his correspondence with the Corinthian congregation, the Apostle appears almost as a psychosomatic physician.

In the debates surrounding Communion, Paul argues that people fall ill because the congregation celebrates Communion in a fundamentally wrong way, because something is wrong with the way people live together in the congregation in Corinth. "For all who eat and drink without discerning the body, eat and drink judgment against themselves. For this reason, many of you are weak and ill, and some have died" (1 Cor. 11:29 f.). This means that a psychosocial conflict has effects even at the somatic level—and it is the wisdom of the lived body, which the Corinthians underestimate, that alerts people to the fact that not all is well in Corinth. Hence, Paul explains to the Corinthians the message their lived bodies express in falling ill. Like a physician, Paul is a hermeneut who makes plain to the patient what the illness is trying to say. It is important to grasp the judging truth in the situation of the illness, which Paul describes as one of crisis. In this sense, the illness presents an opportunity for transformation.

Through illness, psychic and physical, the lived body alerts people to the fact that in the congregation, people lead the wrong kind of lives. Paul critiques the congregation for failing to celebrate Communion properly. Instead of celebrating a communal meal, in which everybody would eat their fill, each eats what they brought themselves, without sharing. This way, some end up drunk while others go hungry. Paul understands the illnesses, which appear to occur in an increased number in the congregation, as a consequence of this false way of celebrating Communion. Interestingly, Paul does not say, "those who eat like this will be judged by God," but rather argues that they "eat and drink judgment against themselves" (1 Cor. 11:29). Ill people are not punished by God. Nevertheless, Paul confronts the Corinthians with the insight that illnesses express the fact that something is wrong, something has gone awry—with me, in my environment, between me and my surroundings. This interpretation of the biblical passage is all the more persuasive once we realize that the terms of illness that Paul uses, *astheneis* and *arrōstoi* (denoting weak and ill people) are mainly used

---

[49] On the following, see Annette Weissenrieder and Gregor Etzelmüller, "Illness and Healing in Christian Traditions," in *Religion and Illness*, ed. Annettte Weissenrieder and Gregor Etzelmüller (Eugene, Ore.: Wipf & Stock, 2016), 263–305; Annette Weissenrieder, "'Darum sind viele körperlich und seelisch Kranke unter euch' (1 Kor 11,29 ff.): Die korinthischen Überlegungen zum Abendmahl im Spiegel antiker Diätetik und der Patristik," in *"Eine gewöhnliche und harmlose Speise"? Von den Entwicklungen frühchristlicher Abendmahlstraditionen*, ed. Judith Hartenstein et al. (Gütersloh: Gütersloher, 2008), 239–68.

in a dietetic connection in the pagan culture of Paul's day. If we read Paul in this context, we can say that the lived body shows a high degree of sensitivity for forms and orders of social coexistence that are detrimental to life.

One important point in this context is that it is not only—not even primarily—the actual perpetrators who fall ill. For those "eating and drinking in an unworthy manner ... obviously had no problems surviving";[50] otherwise Paul would not have had to admonish them. The lived bodies thus react quite differently to grievances in the congregation. There are some who suffer more than others—but in their suffering the truth is revealed that an entire community is caught up in a false kind of life.

In my opinion, it is crucial for our understanding of this text by Paul that we do not understand the illnesses that we encounter in the Corinthian congregation as a punishment by God—contrary to the later reception of this passage. The judgment by God of which Paul speaks is not that members of the Corinthian congregation fall ill and die. God is not a murderer! God's judgment consists in a salutary uncovering of what illnesses, as the organic consequences of a psychosocial conflict, express. The lived body can alert people to the fact that they live a false kind of life; and this is the wisdom of the lived body. Those who attend to their lived bodies in such a way—either in self-critique (1 Cor. 11:31) or because God is making them understand what their lived bodies are trying to say to them—can change their lives, thus being spared from impending ruin (see 1 Cor. 11:32).

To sum up, Paul pursues an attitude to illness that corresponds to Weizsäcker's, who opposed the classic way of thinking about disease that says, "let's get rid of this," with his alternative mindset that responds to illness, "yes, but not in this way." "Saying 'yes' to what the body is trying to communicate, yet making the caveat 'but not in this way' regarding the way the body communicates its message, that is, regarding the way the body has the illness stand in for what it wants to say."[51]

4. The Concrete Destiny of the Individual Person

In the dialogue between medical anthropology and theology, we have detected thus far two insights. First, we have seen that human persons are destined to communicate faith, hope, and love and to build congregations and communities shaped by these attitudes—and to contribute to the building up and preservation of social systems in which justice, mercy, and the search for truth are vital fac-

---

[50] Günter Bornkamm, "Herrenmahl und Kirche bei Paulus," in *Studien zu Antike und Urchristentum: Gesammelte Aufsätze*, vol. 2 (Munich: Kaiser, 1959), 138–76, 170.

[51] Weizsäcker, "Das Problem des Menschen in der Medizin," 369 f.

tors. Second, we are faced with the task of discovering the wisdom of the lived body, as it is presented both in medical anthropology and in biblical traditions. If we are realizing that human destiny of course takes a particular shape for every person, in any situation in life, we have to ask how we can discern our own individual destiny—and how the wisdom of the body can help us by this task. How to discern an individual's destiny has preoccupied philosophers, theologians, and physicians on both sides of the Atlantic, notably in the 1920 s.

To begin with, we can say with Martin Heidegger: in order to recognize my destiny, I must break the spell that "Man" has on me, the uniformity of average life. Instead of asking about their own destiny, people take their cues from the anonymous ordinary person, looking to "the they." Individuals run the risk of mistaking themselves "in listening to the they. This listening must be shattered, that is, the possibility of another kind of hearing that interrupts that listening must be given by Dasein itself. The possibility of such a breach lies in being summoned without any mediation."[52] In this context, Heidegger adopts the concept of the conscience: in order to recognize one's own destiny, we have to distance ourselves from the life plans that others have always already provided and listen to our own conscience. In the conscience, a person is summoned "to its ownmost potentiality-of-being" (263).

Heidegger's philosophy has been called "Protestantism at its nadir of secularization."[53] That makes sense, and it also implies further consequences. Heidegger secularizes the notion that in the end, every individual[54] will be asked by God as their judge how they have made use of the talents they have been given (see Matt. 25:14–30, Luke 19:12–27). Heidegger transforms the expectation that the individual is called out in judgment in such a way that now it is no longer God, but death itself as the "*ownmost* possibility of Dasein" that "individualizes" the person (252).

We can object that natural death does not, of all things, individualize; in equalizing all, death renders people indifferent. Anticipating death, people could just as well recognize that in the end, they will share the lot of all organic life (see Eccl. 3:19 f.)—and draw the conclusion: "Let us eat and drink, for tomorrow

---

[52] Martin Heidegger, *Being and Time*, trans. Joan Stambaugh (Albany: State University of New York Press, 2010), 261. Page numbers in parentheses refer to this work.

[53] Jürgen Habermas, *Philosophical-Political Profiles* (Oxford: Wiley, 2018), 57.

[54] See Friedrich-Wilhelm Marquardt, *Was dürfen wir hoffen, wenn wir hoffen dürften? Eine Eschatologie*, vol. 3 (Gütersloh: Gütersloher, 1996), 304–22, 305: It is not before "their unique encounter with God, face to face, that [people] freely become aware of themselves. Only here they are truly asked about themselves, only here they truly get to know themselves, ceasing to ask for themselves in vain." God calls every individual by their name (Isa. 43:1).

we die" (1 Cor. 15:32). Death only individualizes when perceived as the question what I have made of my life.⁵⁵

Yet Heidegger's secularization effort has particular consequences. Since existence is thrown back onto itself, "Dasein calls itself in conscience," the call of conscience takes place "in the mode of silence."⁵⁶ The call does not have any particular content, but summons me to embrace that which is, my being thrown, as my own choice (275 f.). Conscience loses its critical force and reaffirms that which is already the case.⁵⁷

Alfred North Whitehead similarly prizes the experience of conscience, which he defines like Heidegger in terms of "solitariness."⁵⁸ Presenting his views in 1926, the same year in which Heidegger published *Being and Time*, Whitehead speaks of religious experience. Here, however, God is present as "that element in virtue of which our purposes extend beyond values for ourselves to values for others. He is that element in virtue of which the attainment of such a value for others transforms itself into value for ourselves" (158). God beckons the human person to fulfill possibilities that exceed "our own interests" (ibid.). Precisely in this way, God is "the mirror which discloses to every creature its own greatness" (155). To recognize one's own destiny, a person needs to break the spell of "the they" (*das Man*), in Heidegger's terms, or break the spell of "the they" that is considered sacred; a person needs to break with religious traditions (28 f., 37, 47). Therefore, real greatness does not consist in the conscious choice of that present reality into which the person is thrown, but in the embrace of the new that is in keeping with God's love.⁵⁹ In religious experience,

---

55   Christof Gestrich, *Die menschliche Seele: Hermeneutik ihres dreifachen Weges* (Tübingen: Mohr Siebeck, 2019), 27 f.
56   Ibid., 263, 264; italics removed in both citations.
57   Heidegger basically assumes that, as finite beings, humans do not have enough time to begin something genuinely new. See also Odo Marquard, *Der Einzelne: Vorlesungen zur Existenzphilosophie* (Stuttgart: Reclam, 2013), 234–7. Jewish-Christian tradition objects, however, with its emphasis on new beginnings, for example with Abraham, Moses, and Paul, up to new creation (2 Cor. 5:17). This tradition is articulated in Hannah Arendt's critique of Heidegger's thought on finitude: human persons are "born . . . in order to begin." Arendt, *The Human Condition*, ed. Margaret Canovan, 2nd ed. (Chicago: University of Chicago Press, 2018), 246.
58   Alfred North Whitehead, *Religion in the Making: Lowell Lectures 1926*, 6th ed. (New York: Fordham Press, 2009), 16 f.: "Religion is what the individual does with his own solitariness. ... Thus religion is solitariness; and if you are never solitary, you are never religious" (see also p. 47). In our context, this means the individual has never confronted the question of their destiny. Page numbers in parentheses refer to this work.
59   Whitehead speaks of "love" (75), an increasing "complexity of interrelations" (76), and "harmony" (119).

then, "character is developed" (15). This gives critical force to religious experience: for in religious experience, God "confronts what is actual" in the world "with what is possible for it" (159).

Karl Barth is also among the thinkers who, in the 1920 s, worked with the concept of conscience.[60] Similar to Heidegger, Barth argues that in "conscience I hear my own voice" (486): In my conscience, I am faced with my own existence (*Dasein*), my own self–not, however, my enslaved self that is under the power of "the they" and under the spell of sin; rather, my liberated self, "my own voice as that of the redeemed child of God" (486), who embraces in freedom what God desires: the fulfillment of God's aspirations for his creation. If a person cannot participate in an activity in good conscience, all authorities that seek to rule people run up against their ethical limitations: church and state, but also the demands of one's neighbors (see 483). For that reason, no one can delegate to anyone else the question of what they ought to do. As Heidegger and Whitehead do in their fields, in theological ethics Barth likewise claims that solitary existence is required to recognize what God commands in a particular situation. I have to apprehend myself in order to decide if I can participate in some activity in good conscience.

In distinction from Heidegger, but in remarkable agreement with Whitehead, Barth understands conscience as "a revolutionary principle" (487). Conscience points toward that goal that lies beyond my own self-preservation (see 485); it asks me "whether and how far my conduct, my conduct at this moment, is a forward step, i.e., a step towards the future which is promised me by God's word, the future of the Lord and his lordship over all people and things" (486 f.). Conscience calls on people to fulfill possibilities that are genuinely their own but that exceed what is customary or what has already been achieved (see 487): "hence the disquietude which [conscience] brings into the present, into our natural existence, but truly also into our Christianity, into church and state" (487).

Although Barth appreciates conscience, he also sees the danger that people misunderstand its pronouncements. "Conscience does not err. But we err in our hearing of it" (485). This critical reservation implies that an ethics of conscience cannot be played off against attempts to find moral consensus. "Only cautiously and with restraint, then, do we use what we regard as the voice of our conscience as a criterion to establish genuine authority in relation to the voice of our neighbor" (485). In order to recognize one's own destiny, it is necessary to plumb the depths of solitary existence, to be liberated from the mere convention of "the

---

[60] See Karl Barth, *Ethics*, ed. D. Braun, trans. G. W. Bromiley (Eugene, Ore.: Wipf & Stock, 2013). Barth gave this lecture course in the academic year 1928-29; see further on this text John Webster, *Barth's Moral Theology: Human Action in Barth's Thought* (Edinburgh: T&T Clark, 1998), 57-60. Page numbers in parentheses refer to Barth, *Ethics*.

they," but dialogue with others is also required to discern whether I perceive rightly what my conscience is telling me.[61]

At this point of the historical discourse, a train of thought developed by the physician Viktor von Weizsäcker is particularly pertinent. In his 1928 essay "Krankengeschichte"—either a patient's file or their story—he points out that a person "can stand in their own way."[62] This may be precisely what an illness brings to mind (see 65). The point of the illness would then consist in prompting a biographical change. If this is how we understand disease, patients require a physician not merely for their physical plight. The ill person needs the physician so that that "which takes place in the ill person" can be "led on toward its ultimate destiny" (66f.). The physician's task is partly defined by the patient's autonomy; ultimately, only the patient can discern the ultimate meaning of the illness. "The 'meaning of an illness' can only be realized from the patient's perspective; the physician must not dictate the meaning. For the ill person, the meaning can only be salutary; for the physician, it can only be a plight" (66). The physician's task is to accompany patients on their way toward solitary existence as reflective individuals—though not necessarily as an advocate of what the patient does or says, but as an advocate of the self of the patients, so that it can make its voice heard. Weizsäcker speaks concretely about "the physician and the patient as companions on the way" (65, see 58). Similarly, we could speak of friends, therapists, and pastoral care givers as companions on the way to their partner in dialogue, and here the specific challenge for the physician could be to decode what the body is trying to tell the patient in the illness.

To sum up, individuals who discern their destiny—for example, patients who leave hospital and ask what they need to do to become truly healthy—need to be aware of the danger merely to reproduce in their lives how others in their en-

---

[61] In his late work, Barth continued to maintain this dual necessity. On one hand, he argues: "We should be fools if in making use of our opportunities we did not look for examples and teachers, for comrades and brothers. Those who more or less exactly discover their opportunity and more or less decisively grasp it have always definitely to thank others far away or near who have in some way been able to stimulate, encourage, and equip them to do so, even if only by issuing the warning and deterrent: 'Be a man, and do *not* follow me.'" Barth, *Church Dogmatics* III.4, trans. A. T. Mackay et al. (Edinburgh: T&T Clark, 1961), 585 (trans. altered). On the other hand, however, it stands to reason: "The only result of irresolution is the person of clichés who is characterized by what they think to be impressive or advisable as the average of their fortuitous environment, as the person in the street [*das ... 'Man'*], but who is fundamentally characterized by fear of the isolation and risk without which no one can take their place or grasp their opportunity." Ibid., 586 (trans. altered).

[62] Viktor von Weizsäcker, "Krankengeschichte," 53. Page references in parentheses refer to this article.

vironment live. As individuals, they need to be called out of the crowd; they need to allow themselves to be challenged. Of course, the individual always remains a person in need of relationships. In that sense it is a blessing for human beings to have one person or several who accompany them in the lifelong process of finding their own way and destiny—without patronizing them. The question is how the general destiny of the human person—the communication of faith, love, and hope—can become a concrete reality in one's own biography: what ways are there (for me, in my concrete life situation) to strengthen others in their trust, to help them experience love and have hope?

Here the Christian faith gives precedence to the gospel over against any demand. As every person is created in the image of God according to Genesis 1, and as all members have something to contribute to the building up of the congregation (see 1 Cor. 14:26, in correspondence to the Apostle's teaching on gifts), every single person has a role to play in God's story with humanity.[63] God is faithful in not giving up on anyone, continuing his work also on those who fall short of their destiny and fail to live up to their task.[64] And who could ever assert that they have fully satisfied their responsibility?[65]

Since the communication of faith, hope, and love are meant to gain specific shape in every life, nobody needs to do everything. The destiny of a finite person is always itself finite. The tasks to which one could devote oneself are so manifold that people could give up hope, if they had not been freed to do precisely

---

[63] See Barth, *CD* III.4, p. 575: "The fact that in history even the greatest are obviously only transitory, all of them having their time, coming and then going again, means conversely that in history even the smallest are equally indispensable in their way, having their time too, and not coming or going in vain. After all, what is meant by great or small in real history, that is, not the history that is found in books or newspapers, but history as it stands open to the eyes of God and is sometimes perhaps discerned by his angels? We must reckon with the fact that here again there are connections and determinations which would astonish us if only we could see them" (trans. altered). See also Gestrich, *Die menschliche Seele*, 165 f.

[64] See also Gerhard Sauter, *Das verborgene Leben: Eine theologische Anthropologie* (Gütersloh: Gütersloher, 2011), 41: Someone "may perhaps have forgotten God or think of themselves as forsaken by God—they are and will be so well known to God that every moment of their existence is preserved [*aufgehoben*] in God's memory; God will never forget them. That is to say: God will always and forever be concerned about them and attend to them, care for them; which of course also includes that God holds them accountable."

[65] Even Paul writes: "I am not aware of anything against myself, but I am not thereby acquitted. It is the Lord who judges me" (1 Cor. 4:4).

what they perceive as their particular task here and now.⁶⁶ Life's destiny takes on a specific shape for each individual. The New Testament narratives of Jesus's healing the ill make the point in a profound way: by no means are all the healed people called to follow Jesus and become disciples; Jesus sends a paralytic home whom he healed (Mark 2:12); after exorcizing the unclean spirit from the Gerasene man, Jesus keeps him from joining his group, but gives him the task to proclaim Jesus among his friends and family (Mark 5:18–20). In Mark 10, by contrast, Bartimaeus chooses health by deciding to follow Jesus. Human destiny has a particular shape for each of these who were healed. To communicate faith, hope, and love can mean for some to be called to work in public (with proclamation and discipleship) and to take on leadership roles in social systems; for others, it can mean to find their place and fulfill their function in a more intimate circle and to work among friends, the romantic partner, and the family.

If, in this sense, we ask for the destiny of life that may change within one's biography, we will need to ask, second, which ways are likely to strengthen my hope, my love, and my faith? There is a way to practice self-effacement for the benefit of others that does not even ask this question anymore. Ultimately, this kind of activity makes people ill. The metaphor of the source that was used above in describing a person's temple existence also implies that any body of water that is not consistently fed and replenished will run dry eventually.

This prompts the third question for the right balance: how much can any particular person give without becoming exhausted in the long run? What can he or she tolerate without breaking? It is part of the communication of faith, love, and hope to react with faithfulness to unfaithfulness, with forgiveness to lovelessness, to keep up hope where others can only despair.⁶⁷ Self-effacement always implies a sacrifice of vitality, yet the ultimate sacrifice of vitality is death. A person needs to find the right balance between self-effacement and vitality, again and again. We can experience the joyful discovery that there are forms of self-effacement that also enhance vitality. Yet nothing can simply be taken for granted here, and usually the situation is such that first of all, people need to invest, sacrifice certain opportunities for life and a measure of vitality without knowing for certain that these sacrifices will strengthen their own lives.

---

[66] See Barth, *CD* III.4, 587 f.: "With all the demands which crowd in upon them," people "must know how to give preference to one thing and to set aside another. They must know how to concentrate and therefore how to separate the center from the periphery, or from the many peripheries in question" (trans. altered).

[67] As Immanuel Kant already saw, all of this requires "some sacrifice" of the "pleasures of life." Kant, *Anthropology from a Pragmatic Point of View*, Cambridge Texts in the History of Philosophy, ed. Robert B. Louden and Manfred Kuehn (Cambridge: Cambridge University Press, 2006), 226.

In the process of finding a balance, the lived body has a say as well. Paul was open to the idea that in illness, the body communicates that life is lived in a fundamentally wrong way. This may be the case because of one's own activities or because of one's embedding in a community that fails precisely to strengthen faith, love, and hope. In this sense, a theological anthropology of the body argues for a greater attentiveness to one's own lived body. We can feel it in our own bodies, and see in other people's bodies as well, whether the sacrifice of opportunities of life makes them ill or strengthens their vitality. It would be wise to hear out the wisdom of one's body when discerning the destiny of one's own life.

Psychotherapy, Personality, and the Role of Values

Peter Kirsch

When we think about character formation, ethical education, and values in psychotherapy, the concept of personality immediately comes into focus. Personality means the totality of all temporally stable characteristics of a person, which determine his or her experience and behavior. However, in addition to the traditional personality traits, such as intelligence, extroversion, or openness, attitudes and values are also part of these enduring characteristics. Therefore, when we address people's personalities in psychotherapy, we also have to deal with their values. It is important for the psychotherapeutic process to look at people's values and, in particular, their possibilities for living according to them. Finally, it is also important for us psychotherapists to ask how we want to address the definition or change of our patients' values in the psychotherapeutic process. These are the questions we will deal with in this chapter, but before we discuss them, it is necessary to clarify what we mean by psychotherapy, as this also leads to implications for further considerations.

Definition of Psychotherapy

It is always interesting to ask people how they define psychotherapy. Although all of us may have an implicit concept of psychotherapy in our minds, it seems quite difficult to formulate an explicit definition or to agree on it. In clinical psychology, we start from a concept of psychotherapy that, on one hand, implies that the method is used particularly when people have disorders with disease value, but, on the other hand, also requires agreement on the part of the patient to the concept of disorder and the goals of therapy. In a comprehensive definition, Hans Strotzka has described psychotherapy as

> a deliberate and planned interactional process for influencing behavioral disturbances and states of suffering deemed by consensus to require treatment (preferably between patient, therapist, and reference group), by psychological means (through

communication) mostly verbal, but also averbal, toward a defined goal (symptom minimization and/or structural change in personality) worked out together, if possible, by means of teachable techniques based on a theory of normal and pathological behavior.[1]

In our context, the question of structural change in personality is particularly relevant. If psychotherapy is applied only when a disorder with disease value is present, this is a personality disorder. Furthermore, it is relevant that, according to this definition, psychotherapy must always be consensual, both in terms of the problem and in terms of the goal. Thus, if the goal of psychotherapy is a change in personality structure and associated values, these changes must also be desired by the patients themselves. A paternalistic approach, in which the therapist dictates the goals of therapy, is thus questionable. However, here we encounter the problem that personality disorders are less amenable to psychotherapeutic treatment than other mental illnesses.

Personality Disorders

Personality disorders are understood to be a persistent pattern of individuals' experience and behavior that noticeably deviates from social expectations. The pattern leads to repeated or enduring psychosocial and interpersonal crises. While personality disorders can have very different manifestations, ranging from very withdrawn, distrustful, or anxious persons to very quick-tempered, emotionally unstable, or antisocial individuals, what they all have in common is that the disorder is ego-syntonic; that is, the affected individual identifies with their own personality. Moreover, what the disorders also have in common—and this is a direct consequence both of this ego-syntonia and of the fact that it is a stable pattern of experience and behavior—is that they are resistant to any form of change. Those affected therefore initially also show little motivation to allow any changes at all.

If we assume, however, that psychotherapy can take place only if those affected by a mental disorder see the problem themselves and want to change it, the question naturally arises as to why people with a personality disorder should seek psychotherapy at all. They do so primarily because of the aforementioned psychosocial or interpersonal crises to which these individuals are repeatedly exposed. Their own well-being suffers massively if, due to their personality

---

[1] Hans Strotzka, "Was ist Psychotherapie [What is psychotherapy]?," in Hans Strotzka, ed., *Psychotherapie: Grundlagen, Verfahren, Indikationen* [Psychotherapy: basics, methods, indications], 2nd ed. (Munich: Urban & Schwarzenberg, 1978), 3–6. Translation by the author.

structure, they repeatedly clash with their environment. Thus, even people with a narcissistic personality structure—who actually think they are great and special and usually recognize problems only in their fellow human beings—repeatedly find their way to a psychotherapist when they develop depression, for example, due to relationship problems.

Interaction problems can often be traced back to a discrepancy between one's own values and goals. People's values and goals are closely interwoven with their basic needs. If one follows Klaus Grawe,[2] people have four different basic needs in common, which they have in different strengths: (1) the need for orientation and control, (2) the need for pleasure and avoidance of displeasure, (3) the need for attachment, and (4) the need for self-esteem. Depending on the characteristics of one's personality, there may be a contradiction between different basic needs, which then also leads to dissonance and suffering, even in people with ego-syntonic personality disorder. Thus, one can well imagine that in a person with a narcissistic personality structure, the need for self-worth and the need for attachment come into conflict when the people closest to the narcissist may no longer appreciate his or her constant proclamations of grandiosity. People with an anxious-avoidant or even obsessive-compulsive personality structure have great difficulty reconciling the very strong need for orientation and control with the need for pleasure, since the constant controlling must lead to a loss of reinforcers. According to Grawe, the goal of psychotherapy is therefore to achieve a dissonance-free state, in which all basic needs can be satisfied to a sufficient extent without interfering with the satisfaction of other basic needs. In order to achieve such a state, psychotherapy must try to work with the affected person on his or her values and goals and find out how these can be brought into harmony.

Values and Goals in Psychotherapy

In psychotherapy we understand values as points of orientation for one's life. Thus, they are not to be understood in the sense of normative values that a society must agree upon in order to live together prosperously, but they represent factual values[3] that are represented or expressed in concrete patterns of behavior. Of course, factual values can go together with normative values, and at least in the case of universal values, such as humanity or justice, this is the case for most people. Psychotherapeutically, however, it does not really matter at first how the individual's values are assessed by society. This understanding of val-

---

[2] Klaus Grawe, *Psychological Therapy* (Göttingen: Hogrefe & Huber Publishers, 2004).
[3] Charlotte Malachowski Bühler, *Values in Psychotherapy* (Glencoe, Ill.: The Free Press, 1962).

ues shows again their close relation to personality, which also manifests itself in the experience and behavior of the individual. Here, too, the direct connection between values and goals is manifest, since the values of people define their goals and substantially modulate their motivation to show goal-directed behavior. In this understanding, values represent the prerequisite for a self-determined life and the perception of one's own actions as effective.[4]

As already described in the context of basic needs, human suffering is regularly observed when people do not live in accordance with their values and thus do not achieve the goals defined for themselves. However, it must be noted repeatedly that people find it extremely difficult to clearly define their values and, thus, their goals. Psychotherapy therefore has the task of helping people not only to live according to their values, but also to first identify their values or, if this is not possible, to redefine them. Values must also be questioned if they are in competition with other goals and thus make a dissonance-free life difficult.

Difficulties always arise in psychotherapy, however, when the goals of therapists and patients or clients do not coincide. It is a fact, sometimes difficult for therapists to learn, that psychotherapeutic changes can be achieved only if the patients agree with the goals of the therapy.[5]

In summary, it can be stated at this point that psychotherapy addressing changes of personality structure is successful when it helps people to recognize and become aware of or define their basic needs, values, and resulting goals for action. In this context, the perspective of acceptance and commitment therapy (ACT) can be very helpful in distinguishing between approach and avoidance goals. It is primarily the "approach" goals that enable us to live according to our needs and values and to perceive ourselves as self-efficient and successful individuals. At this point, however, the therapist is really only a coach who helps the patient to define his values and goals and to find out what he has to change in order to live according to the values and achieve the goals. Of course, changes can be made by changing behaviors that stand in the way of achieving goals, or by questioning one's values, which may be in conflict with other basic needs, values, or goals. Thus, psychotherapy itself, although it focuses on values, remains value-free, because it does not evaluate the values of the individual. This does not mean, of course, that psychotherapy cannot also consist of consciously

---

[4] Self-efficacy itself is also in turn an important determinant of the success of psychotherapeutic treatment. Fostering an individual's expectation that he or she has an impact on his or her own life or can even change his or her life situation represents an important efficacy factor of psychotherapy.

[5] In addition, in my view, it is equally important that patients understand why a therapeutic method serves to achieve the goal, but since this chapter is supposed to be about general aspects of psychotherapy, all methodological aspects are excluded.

questioning the values—for example, when they are diametrically opposed to the needs and values of the patient's social environment—but the ultimate decision about the definition of goals and values is always left to the patient or client. This leads us to the final question, namely, to what extent psychotherapy may play a role in ethical education, that is, in shaping or defining a person's values.

Does Psychotherapy Have an Educational Function?

This question has two aspects. The first question is to what extent psychotherapy is obliged to teach ethical values and motivate people to live according to the values agreed upon in our society, or even to induce a change in behavior that many people consider necessary.[6] The second question is to what extent psychotherapy can succeed when the psychotherapist is tasked with working with his or her patient or client on goals that contradict the psychotherapist's own values.

The first question has actually already been answered above: psychotherapy cannot have an educational mission if the patient's autonomy and self-determination are taken seriously. Changing values makes sense only if their content is the reason for the individual's suffering. And, of course, living by values that are not shared by one's environment can lead to suffering, and reflection and questioning of such values can certainly be a meaningful part of psychotherapy. We also know that sense-making is an important resilience factor that enables us to go through life in a healthy way, so addressing positive or even religious values can be quite helpful. However, all such changes in values can be based only on the needs of the patient or client, not on the values of the therapist.

Basically, one can indeed state that in our modern pluralistic societies, the acceptance of different values is very high, so that only a few people will formulate values and goals in the context of psychotherapy that are consensually considered unacceptable in our society. Furthermore, in purely pragmatic terms, one could also assume that most people who hold such values are rather unlikely to accept psychotherapeutic help. However, the second question touched upon remains relevant, because a therapist cannot be expected to help a person live according to values or achieve goals that are diametrically opposed to the therapist's own values. Even if one were to overlook such ethical and moral concerns, one cannot imagine that therapy can be successful when the therapist pursues goals for his patient that the therapist himself deeply rejects. In this respect, psychotherapy does indeed reach its limits where people define goals that are

---

[6] Such a discussion is currently being held in the context of the climate crisis, where there are indeed voices that see it as the task of psychotherapy to initiate behavioral changes in people so that they behave in a more climate-friendly way.

contrary to the fundamental values of our society or of the therapist. However, most people come to psychotherapy with the desire to better implement their positive values in their lives, and here psychotherapy can be an important contributor that allows us to live well and in harmony together in society.

Contributors

Karla Alex is Research Associate at the Section for Translational Medical Ethics, National Center for Tumor Diseases (NCT), Heidelberg University Hospital.

Dr. Beate Ditzen is Professor of Medical Psychology and Psychotherapy and Director of the Institute for Medical Psychology at Heidelberg University Hospital.

Dr. Gregor Etzelmüller is Professor of Systematic Theology at the University of Osnabrück.

Dr. Ruth M. Farrell is Associate Professor of Surgery and Vice Chair of Clinical Research at the Women's Health Institute, The Cleveland Clinic, Ohio.

Dr. Anthony Ho is Professor and Director Emeritus of the Department of Internal Medicine: Hematology, Oncology, and Rheumatology, Heidelberg University Hospital.

Dr. Peter Kirsch is Professor and Head of the Department of Clinical Psychology, Central Institute of Mental Health, University of Mannheim.

Dr. Pavlina Lenga is Doctor of Medicine at the University Clinic for Neurosurgery, Heidelberg.

Dr. Thorsten Moos is Professor of Systematic Theology (Ethics) at the University of Heidelberg.

Dr. Karen Nolte is Professor and Director of the Institute of History and Ethics of Medicine at the University of Heidelberg.

Dr. Stephen Pickard, a retired Anglican bishop, is Professor Emeritus and former Director of the Australian Centre for Christianity and Culture, Charles Sturt University, Canberra.

Dr. Nadia Primc is Research Associate at the Institute of History and Ethics of Medicine, Medical Faculty, University of Heidelberg.

Dr. Giovanni Rubeis is Professor of Biomedical and Public Health Ethics, Karl Landsteiner University, Krems.

Dr. Christian P. Schaaf is University Professor in Human Genetics and Managing Director of the Institute of Human Genetics at the University of Heidelberg.

Dr. Christine Thomas is Associate Professor and Head of the Department of Geriatric Psychiatry at the Stuttgart Clinic of Psychiatry and Psychotherapy.

Dr. Dr. Günter Thomas is Chair of Ethics and Fundamental Theology at Bochum University, Germany, and Research Associate at the Faculty of Theology, Stellenbosch University, South Africa.

Dr. Andreas Unterberg is Professor and Head of the Department of Adult and Pediatric Neurosurgery, Heidelberg University Hospital.

Dr. Dr. Michael Welker is Senior Professor of Systematic Theology and Director of the FIIT–Research Center for International and Interdisciplinary Theology at the University of Heidelberg.

Dr. Dr. Eva C. Winkler is Professor and Director of the Research Group "Ethics and Patient-Oriented Care in Oncology" at the National Center for Tumor Diseases (NCT), University of Heidelberg.

Dr. Dr. John Witte Jr. is the Robert W. Woodruff Professor of Law, McDonald Distinguished Professor of Religion, and Faculty Director of the Center for the Study of Law and Religion at Emory University.